INTERMITTENT FASTING AND KETO DIET

THIS BOOK INCLUDES: "
Intermittent Fasting + Keto Diet"

By David Clark

GW00455237

INTERMITTENT FASTING

Conclusion: 87

KETO

Chapter 7: Smoothies Recipes 211

Conclusion 220

INTERMITTENT FASTING

55 Recipes For Intermittent Fasting and Healthy Rapid Weight Loss

Introduction:

Intermittent fasting is an example of eating that alternates between times of fasting, normally devouring just water, and non-fasting, generally eating anything a person needs regardless of how stuffing. In the evening time, a person can eat anything he needs for 24 hours and fast for the following 24 hours. This way to deal with weight control is by all accounts upheld by science, just as strict and social practices throughout the planet. Followers of Intermittent fasting guarantee that this training is an approach to turn out to be more careful about food.

Also, an Intermittent fasting diet is somewhat unique from ordinary fasting. This kind of transient fasting doesn't decrease fat-consuming chemicals. Truth be told, logical exploration has shown that the specific inverse occurs and you will begin expanding the movement of fat-consuming catalysts.

An incredible part of Intermittent fasting is that there isn't a lot of exertion included. You can carry on with life, go out to eat, still have your favorite food sources and a periodic treat. The weight loss can be quick or consistent relying upon how you approach it. You can be as severe or loose about your eating as you need and still get more fit. Eating this way is useful for breaking levels as well.

To benefit from Intermittent fasting, you need to fast for at any rate 16 hours. At 16 hours or more, a portion of the stunning advantages of Intermittent fasting kicks in. A simple method to do this is to just skip breakfast each day. This is in reality extremely solid, however, many people will try to disclose to you in any case. By skipping breakfast, you are permitting your body to go into a caloric shortfall, which will enormously build the measure of fat you can consume and the weight you can lose.

Since your body isn't caught up with processing the food you ate, it has the opportunity to zero in on consuming your fat stores for energy and for purifying and detoxifying your body. If you think that it's hard to skip breakfast, you can rather skip a meal, even though I track down this considerably more troublesome.

It truly doesn't make any difference, yet the objective is to broaden the timeframe you spend fasting and loss the measure of time you spend eating. If you have a meal at 6 PM and don't eat until 10 the following morning, you have refrained for 16 hours. Longer is better, however, you can see some beautiful extraordinary changes from every day 16 hours fast.

Chapter: 1 Breakfast

1: Healthy Tuna Mornay

A better smooth fish pasta heat loaded with heaps of vegetables and surprisingly some mysterious beans. The ideal family-accommodating pasta dish that works for babies and adults. There are alternatives to make this gluten-free, lactose-free, or even dairy-free.

Ingredients:

- 1 block chicken stock
- Salt and pepper
- 4 tbsp. Parmesan cheddar
- 2 tsp lemon juice
- 1.25 cups light coconut milk
- 1.5 tbsp. whole meal flour
- 1 tbsp. margarine
- 1 tsp coconut oil
- 425 g canned fish in spring water
- 1/4 cup whole meal breadcrumbs
- 1 cup frozen or tinned peas or corn or veg of decision

Method:

- Preheat oven to 180C.
- Channel fish and spot in a blending bowl.
- Add corn to the bowl and blend well.
- Season with salt and pepper.
- Cook cubed onions in coconut oil until delicate.
- Add onions to fish blend, mix well.

- Add spread to frypan and soften.
- Pour in coconut milk and gradually add the flour, whisking continually to stay away from knots.
- Add 3 tbsp. of the Parmesan cheddar and the lemon juice.
- Disintegrate the stock shape and sprinkle over the top, then add prepared to taste.
- Blend well.
- Pour sauce over the fish combination and mix until very much consolidated.
- Tip into stove confirmation dishes – it is possible that one huge dish, or personal dishes.
- Combine as one whole meal breadcrumb and the leftover Parmesan cheddar and sprinkle over the fish blend.
- Cook in the oven for 25 minutes and afterward grill for a further 5-10 mins until brilliant earthy colored on top.
- Fill in with no guarantees or with steamed greens, pasta, salad, or rice.

2: Sweet Potato & Black Bean Burrito

Sound Sweet Potato and Black Bean Burrito are loaded down with such a lot of goodness. Your number one tortilla or wrap is loaded up with chime pepper, yam, black beans, avocado, and earthy colored rice for a nutritious dish with stunning flavor. These are normally gluten-free (contingent upon the tortilla) veggie-lover burritos that make an astonishing breakfast, lunch, or dinner that is prepared in less than 30 minutes.

Ingredients:

- fine grain ocean salt
- 1 big red onion, cut
- avocado oil (I utilized Primal Kitchen)
- ground chipotle powder
- 4–6 burrito estimated tortillas
- hot sauce or salsa, whenever wanted (I love a tomatillo one with these!!)
- 1 large or 2 little yams, slashed into 1/2" blocks (no compelling reason to strip, simply wash them well!!)
- 1 15-ounce container of black beans, flushed and depleted

Method:

- Preheat stove to 400 F.
- On a material-lined dish, toss red onions and yams with enough avocado oil to cover and a liberal measure of salt and some chipotle powder.
- Prepare for 20-30 minutes, tossing a couple of times, until yams are effectively penetrated with a fork and onions are earthy colored (whatever's cooking excessively, move more to the middle!).
- Add the black beans to the oven and toss to blend.
- Warm tortillas for 30 seconds on each side to make them flexible (this is too essential to keep them from breaking when you try to overlap them!) then do a line of the black bean and yam combination down the center.
- Add hot sauce if utilizing. Crease in sides and roll. As far as I might be concerned, this made 5 burritos, yet

it'll shift dependent on the size of your tortillas. Wrap burritos in foil, and hold up!

- To plan, microwave, or utilize a toaster to warm when prepared to eat.

3: Pb and J Overnight Oats

These PB&J Overnight Oats are a definitive make-ahead breakfast that will keep you powered and empowered throughout the day with whole-grain moved oats, chia seeds, peanut butter, and jam. Make your oats with this natively constructed Chia Seed Jam and add your number one fresh organic product. Overnight cereal is a steady staple in my morning meal routine since it is something I can prepare early and I realize will keep me full throughout the morning.

Ingredients:

- 1 cup moved oats
- 1 tablespoon chia seeds
- 1 cup unsweetened almond milk
- 1/2 tablespoon maple syrup
- 1 tablespoon jam or jelly
- 2 tablespoons rich peanut butter

Method:

- Spot all ingredients short the jam in a glass Tupperware and blend.
- Cover and let sit in the cooler for at any rate 2 hours or overnight.
- In the morning, twirl in some jam and appreciate cold.

4: Porridge with Apple and Cinnamon

Porridge is consistently an extraordinary method to begin the day, regardless of whether you're an infant, youngster, or grown-up. My apple and cinnamon porridge is pressed brimming with flavor. You can eat it also, or jazz it up for certain additional ingredients - I like walnut nuts and poppy seeds. My variant is appropriate for vegetarians; however, you can utilize your preferred milk.

Ingredients:

- 2 tbsp. honey
- 1 section moved oats to 2 sections of milk
- 1 apple
- Touch of salt
- Small bunch toasted walnuts, generally chopped

Method:

- Measure the porridge in a little glass then add it to a little sauce container with twice the milk.
- Spot the pan on medium-high heat and bring to the bubble, then turn off the heat.
- Add a touch of salt and mix reliably until you have a thick, velvety blend, this will take about 8-10minutes.
- Mesh the apple and mix half of it into the porridge, then add the cinnamon and honey and blend well.
- Serve the porridge in a bowl then top it with the remainder of the ground apple, some more cinnamon, and honey.
- Sprinkle the toasted walnuts on top, it's a decent option to add some virus milk over the top if you like.

5: Greek Chickpea Waffles

Waffles are a morning meal staple which is as it should be. They're regularly fleecy, sweet, and covered in margarine— who could want anything more? However, in case you're attempting to go for something somewhat better (and would prefer not to hit your daily calorie quantity just after breakfast), choosing appetizing waffles can make breakfast in a hurry quite a lot more stimulating.

Ingredients:

- 1/2 tsp. heating pop
- 3/4 c. chickpea flour
- 1/2 tsp. salt
- 6 huge eggs
- 3/4 c. plain 2% Greek yogurt
- Cucumbers, parsley, yogurt, tomatoes, scallion, and lemon juice, for serving

Method:

- Heat stove to 200°F. Set a wire rack over a rimmed heating sheet and spot it on the stove. Heat waffle iron per bearings.
- In a big bowl, preparing pop, whisk together flour, and salt.
- In a little bowl, whisk together yogurt and eggs.
- Mix wet ingredients into dry ingredients.
- Gently cover waffle iron with nonstick cooking shower and, in clumps, drop ¼ to ½ cup player into each segment of iron and cook until brilliant earthy colored, 4 to 5 minutes.
- Move to the stove and keep warm. Rehash with the leftover player.
- Serve finished off with cucumbers, tomatoes, and scallion threw with olive oil, pepper, salt, and parsley.
- Shower with yogurt blended in with lemon juice.

Firm quesadillas loaded up with beans, ringer pepper, sautéed onions, avocado, and bunches of cheddar. These avocado black bean quesadillas are filling and make an extraordinary vegan feast as well. They make an extraordinary breakfast and are very filling as well!

Ingredients:

- 4 delicate flour or corn tortillas
- 1 avocado, hollowed, stripped, and cut into pieces
- 4 ounces Manchego cheddar, cut
- 16 canned or jolted jalapeño cuts

Method:

- Get out 1 tortilla on a work surface.
- Spot about a fourth of the cheddar on one half, not very close to the edge so the cheddar won't soften out as it cooks.
- Top cheddar with a fourth of the avocado and four jalapeño cuts.
- Overlap tortilla fifty-fifty over filling to frame a half-circle.
- Heat a grill container or oven over medium heat.
- Slide uncooked quesadilla onto the oven.
- Crunch down with a weight or simply press momentarily with a spatula.
- Cook 1 moment, then flip the quesadilla and flame broil brief more or until cheddar is liquefied.
- Move the quesadilla to a cutting board and cut it into 6 wedges. Serve right away. Rehash with residual ingredients. Makes 24 wedges.

This recipe for veggie lover fish tacos is loaded with flavor yet, however, so natural to plan! There's no untidy twofold digging of these children, a too basic one bowl fish 'n chips-style hitter is all you need to get incredibly firm vegetarian "fish" bits ideal for ingredient your Baja fish taco wanting. These veggie-lover fish tacos are stunningly presented with an avocado plate of mixed greens and my blackberry margaritas.

Ingredients:

- 2/3 cup water
- 1/2 cup panko breadcrumbs
- 2 teaspoons nori powder (discretionary, for an 'off-putting' taste)
- 1/2 teaspoon salt
- 2 tablespoons lemon juice
- 1/2 cup flour
- 1 (14 ounces) bundle firm or extra firm tofu, depleted and squeezed
- 2 tablespoons soy sauce or tamari
- 1 tablespoon cornstarch

Rich Lime Slaw:

- 2 tablespoons lime juice
- 1/3 cup veggie-lover mayo of decision
- 1/2 teaspoon stew powder
- 1/4 teaspoon ground cumin
- 1/4 teaspoon salt
- 1/2 teaspoon garlic powder
- 4–5 cups finely destroyed cabbage

Method:

- Preheat the stove to 450 degrees F.
- Make the tofu fish sticks: In one bowl, combine as one the soy sauce, lemon juice, and nori powder.
- In another bowl, whisk together the flour and cornstarch, then gradually race in the water to make a play.
- Put the excess breadcrumbs and salt in a third bowl.
- Cut the tofu into finger-like strips, then plunge into the lemon bowl, the flour player, and finely the panko.
- Spot on a lubed preparing sheet and proceed with the remainder of the tofu.
- Heat for 10 minutes, then flip and cook an extra 8 minutes, or until brilliant earthy colored and fresh.
- While the tofu is cooking, whisk together the elements for the slaw in a big bowl: the mayo, lime squeeze, and preparing.
- Taste, adding more flavors/salt depending on the situation.
- Then include the cabbage and throw well, proceeding to throw the cabbage will cover the cabbage and begin to separate it so it's simpler to eat.
- Warm the tortillas, then partition the tofu onto the tortillas and top with slaw.
- Spurt with all the fresher lime juice, whenever wanted, and appreciate!

8: Peach Berry Smoothie

Smoothies are one of my #1-morning meals or evening jolts of energy (so extraordinary when you live someplace blistering!). I love that there are in a real sense unlimited blends and in its single direction my children will cheerfully eat (drink?) their veggies and pack in some extra organic product. This blueberry peach smoothie dairy-free, normally improved and so delightful on account of delicious peaches and blueberries.

Ingredients:

- 1/2 cup almond milk or most loved juice
- 3/4 cup Driscoll's Blueberries
- 1 Tbsp. ground flaxseeds
- 1/2 cup non-fat plain Greek yogurt
- 2 Tablespoons honey
- 1 little peach, generally slashed, or 1/2 cup frozen peaches
- 3 Ounces ice solid shapes (not required if utilizing frozen peaches)

Method:

- Mix blueberries, peach, almond milk, flaxseeds, honey, yogurt, and ice in a blender until pureed and smooth, mixing a few times.
- Serve right away.

Beginning your day with a sound Green Breakfast Smoothie is an incredible method to get empowered and feel great. This one is sound and delicious … a triumphant combo. Drinking this daily smoothie is the thing that assisted me with getting the body and energy to do some unimaginable things. Most smoothies are made with simply foods grown from the ground, which is high in sugar and can cause aggravation. A green smoothie, then again, is made with fruit, plant-based fluid, and verdant greens.

Ingredients:

- 1 huge mango, frozen
- 1 green apple, cored
- 1/2 English cucumber
- 6 little leaves of romaine (or 3 modest bunches of spinach)
- 1/2 lemon, stripped and cultivated
- 2 celery stems
- cold sifted water to mix (around 2 cups)

Method:

- Spot everything into a fast blender and mix until smooth.
- Serve and appreciate right away.

10: Chicken Breasts with Avocado Tapenade

It's another best recipe for irregular fasting referenced in the morning meal list. You can make it easy and within a short time. It's truly tasty and everybody will like it.

Ingredients:

- 1/2 teaspoon salt
- 1 tablespoon ground lemon strip
- 4 boneless skinless chicken bosom parts
- 5 tablespoons fresh lemon juice, isolated
- 1 teaspoon olive oil, partitioned
- 2 tablespoons olive oil, partitioned
- 1 garlic clove, finely cleaved
- 1/4 teaspoon ground black pepper
- 2 garlic cloves, cooked and pounded
- 1/2 teaspoon ocean salt
- 1 medium tomato, cultivated and finely cleaved
- 1/4 teaspoon fresh ground pepper
- 1/4 cup little green pimento-stuffed olives, meagerly cut
- 2 tablespoons fresh basil leaves, finely cut
- 3 tablespoons escapades, washed
- 1 big avocado, split, hollowed, stripped, and finely cleaved

Method:

- In a sealable plastic pack, consolidate chicken and marinade of the lemon strip, 2 tablespoons lemon juice, garlic, 2 tablespoons olive oil, salt, and pepper.
- Seal sack and refrigerate for 30 minutes.
- In a bowl, whisk together the leftover 3 tablespoons lemon juice, staying 1/2 teaspoons olive oil, ocean salt, simmered garlic, and fresh ground pepper.
- Blend in tomato, green olives, escapades, basil, and avocado; put in a safe spot.
- Eliminate chicken from the sack and dispose of marinade.

- Grill over medium-hot coals for 4 to 5 minutes for every side or to the ideal level of doneness.
- Present with Avocado Tapenade.

11: Meal Club Tilapia Parmesan

This is a very basic dish, so several excessively basic side dishes are all you need. These Sautéed Green Beans with Cherry Tomatoes. I would simply keep it simple. I think one normal misinterpretation of this recipe is that it ought to be fresh. "Crusted" in this case simply implies that it is shrouded in Parmesan.

Ingredients:

- black pepper
- 1 scramble hot pepper sauce
- 2 tablespoons lemon juice
- 2 lbs. tilapia filets
- 1/2 cup ground parmesan cheddar
- 3 tablespoons mayonnaise
- 4 tablespoons margarine, room temperature
- 3 tablespoons finely slashed green onions
- 1/4 teaspoon dried basil
- 1/4 teaspoon preparing salt

Method:

- Preheat oven to 350 degrees.
- In a buttered 13-by-9-inch heating dish or jellyroll container, lay filets in a solitary layer.
- Do not stack filets.
- Brush top with juice.
- In a bowl consolidate cheddar, margarine, mayonnaise, onions, and flavors.

- Blend well in with a fork.
- Prepare fish in preheated oven for 10 to 20 minutes or until fish simply begins to piece.
- Spread with cheddar combination and prepare until brilliant earthy colored, about 5minutes.
- Heating time will rely upon the thickness of the fish you use.
- Watch fish intently with the goal that it doesn't overcook.
- Makes 4 servings.
- Note: This fish can likewise be made in an oven.
- Sear 3 to 4 minutes or until practically done.
- Add cheddar and sear another 2 to 3 minutes or until sautéed.

12: Broccoli Dal Curry

Broccoli Curry is a simple and sound sauce or curry dish that can be presented with hot phulkas or steamed rice. This lovely green vegetable is a storage facility of nutrients and minerals. This recipe safeguards every one of the first supplements of broccoli since it doesn't overcook the broccoli florets.

Ingredients:

- 1 – Potato
- 1 - Broccoli
- 1 - Onion
- 1/2 tsp - Ginger and Garlic glue
- 1/4 cup - Cut Corn
- 1/2 tsp - Dhania Jeera powder
- 1/2 tsp - Urad dal
- Salt and Red Chili powder to taste
- 1 squeeze - Turmeric powder

- 1/2 tsp - Mustard seeds
- 4 tsp - Oil

Method:

- Cut the broccoli into little pieces and cook in the microwave for 6 minutes.
- Heat oil in a container and add urad dal, mustard seeds and fry them to a brilliant brown tone.
- Cleave the onion and potato into pieces, add it to the above blend and fry till the potato is bubbled.
- Add to the abovementioned, ginger and garlic glue, dhania and jeera powder, a little turmeric powder, and if you need 1/2 tsp garam masala.
- Add the cooked broccoli pieces alongside slicing corn and salt to taste and red stew powder, and cook it for 5 minutes.
- Your broccoli curry is fit to be presented with one or the other rice or chapatti.

13: Pie Maker Zucchini Slice Muffins

Here is another best recipe for your morning meal. You can undoubtedly make this recipe at your home. It's an astonishing recipe that everybody will very much want to have.

Ingredients:

- 200g yam, stripped, coarsely ground
- 80ml (1/3 cup) extra virgin olive oil
- 2 medium zucchini (about 300g), managed, coarsely ground
- 5 eggs, delicately whisked
- 150g (1 cup) self-rising flour

- 100g (1 cup) Perfect Italiano Perfect Bakes cheddar (mozzarella, cheddar, and parmesan)

Method:

- Heat 1 tablespoon of the oil in a medium non-stick oven over medium-high heat.
- Add the yam and cook, mixing periodically, for 5 minutes or until mollified. Move to a big bowl.
- Add the zucchini, flour, cheddar, egg, and remaining oil.
- Season well and mix to join.
- Preheat the pie producer.
- Fill the pie producer openings with a yam blend.
- Close, cook for 8 minutes.
- Rehash with the excess blend.
- Serve warm or cold.

14: Simmered Broccoli with Lemon-Garlic and Toasted Pine Nuts

So natural thus great. Simmered broccoli with lemon zing, pine nuts, and a sprinkle of Parmesan, on the table in minutes with a little prep work. You'll cherish how the fresh, dynamic broccoli gets punched up with fiery stew chips and a solid hit of lemon juice, in addition to the stunning, rich kind of toasted pine nuts.

Ingredients:

- 2 tablespoons olive oil
- 1-pound broccoli florets
- 2 tablespoons unsalted spread
- 1 teaspoon minced garlic
- Salt and freshly ground black pepper
- 1/2 teaspoon ground lemon zing

- 2 tablespoons pine nuts, toasted
- 1 to 2 tablespoons fresh lemon juice

Method:

- Preheat oven to 500°F.
- In a big bowl, throw the broccoli with the oil and salt, and pepper to taste.
- Mastermind the florets in a solitary layer on a preparing sheet and meal, turning once, for 12 minutes, or until simply delicate.
- In the meantime, in a little pot, soften the spread over medium heat.
- Add the garlic and lemon zing and heat, blending, for around 1 moment.
- Let cool somewhat and mix in the lemon juice.
- Spot the broccoli in a serving bowl, pour the lemon margarine over it and throw to cover.
- Dissipate the toasted pine nuts over the top and serve.

15: The Easiest Hard-Boiled Eggs

Hard-bubbled eggs are an extraordinary food to have available as their uses are so adaptable. In addition to the fact that they are too delectable all alone, yet they're incredible in sandwiches, cleaved up on a salad, and the establishment for all devilled eggs. The secret to incredible hard-bubbled eggs isn't over-cooking them, which can leave a dim ring around the yolk and make their surface somewhat rubbery.

Ingredients:

- 1 tbsp. Sea salt
- 4 cups Water (or enough to cover eggs in the oven)
- 8 big Egg (or any number you need)

- 1 tbsp. Apple juice vinegar (or white if not paleo)

Method:

- Spot your crude eggs in a medium pan and cover with at least 2 creeps of cold water.
- Add 1 tablespoon of salt.
- Spot the dish over high heat until it arrives at a bubble.
- Mood killer heat, cover, and let it sit for 13 minutes.
- After precisely 13 minutes, eliminate the eggs from the dish and spot them in an ice-water shower and let them cool for five minutes.
- Cautiously break the eggs shells (ensuring most of the shell is broken).
- Delicately start eliminating the shells. The ice-water shower will "stun" the film in the middle of the egg-white and the eggshell, releasing the shell and permitting you to strip it off in almost one piece.
- Depending on the situation, you can plunge the egg (as you are stripping it) all through the water to eliminate any bits of the shell.
- Serve promptly, use in a recipe, or store in your fridge for three days.

16: Turkish Egg Breakfast

Turkish eggs recipe creates the ideal breakfast. Turkish Menemen Recipe is an incredibly delectable breakfast recipe. Summer tomatoes and green peppers consolidate with eggs in a container to simplify this, fast, and very yummy supper.

Ingredients:

- 2 tsp lemon juice
- 1 garlic clove, squashed

- 200g/7oz Greek-style plain yogurt
- 1 tsp ocean salt pieces
- 2 tbsp. unsalted spread
- 1 tsp Aleppo pepper
- 1 tbsp. extra virgin olive oil
- 2 huge free-roaming eggs, ice chest cold
- thick sourdough toast, to serve
- barely any fronds fresh dill, cleaved

Method:

- Top a pan off to 4cm/1½in profound with water and bring to the bubble.
- Spot the yogurt into a heatproof bowl sufficiently big to sit over the oven and mix in the garlic and salt.
- Spot the bowl over the oven, ensuring the base doesn't contact the water.
- Mix until it arrives at the internal heat level and has the consistency of softly whipped twofold cream.
- Mood killer the heat, leaving the bowl over the dish.
- Dissolve the spread tenderly in a different little pan until it is simply starting to turn hazelnut-earthy colored.
- Turn the heat off, then mix in the oil, trailed by the Aleppo pepper, and put in a safe spot.
- Fill a wide, lidded pot with 4cm/1½in water and spot over medium heat. Line a big plate with kitchen paper.
- Break the initial egg into a little fine-network sifter suspended over a little bowl, then lift and twirl delicately for around 30 seconds, giving the watery piece of the white trickle access to the bowl; dispose of.

- Delicately tip the egg into a little cup or ramekin and pour 1 teaspoon of lemon juice onto it, focusing on the white. Rehash with the subsequent egg.
- At the point when the poaching water is simply beginning to stew, tenderly slide in the eggs, one on each side of the oven.
- Turn the heat directly down so there is no development in the water, and poach the eggs for 3–4 minutes, until the whites are set and the yolks still runny.
- Move the eggs to the lined plate utilizing an opened spoon.
- Separation the warm, rich yogurt between two shallow dishes, top each with a poached egg, pour over the peppery spread, dissipate the slashed dill on top and eat with the toast.

17: Veggie lover Coconut Kefir Banana Muffins

Simple to make, with simple ingredients, these clammy vegetarian banana biscuits are a pleasant base for fruit, nuts, and even chocolate chips. Blend and match your number one extra items to make your form utilizing our recipe as a format. Eat these biscuits warm with vegetarian margarine and natural product for breakfast, with nut spread for a protein-stuffed bite, or with a scoop of veggie lover frozen yogurt for a simple and tasty pastry.

Ingredients:

- 1 cup oats
- 1 tsp. vanilla concentrate
- 3 bananas
- 3 tbsp. maple syrup
- 1 cup coconut milk

- 1 tsp. heating pop
- 2 tsp. heating powder
- ½ cup slashed walnuts
- 2 tbsp. chipped or destroyed coconut
- 1 ¼ cups whole wheat flour + ¼ cup coconut flour

Method:

- Preheat oven to 350.
- Line 12 biscuit tins with papers. In a medium blending bowl, blend oats, flour(s), heating pop, and preparing powder.
- In a different bowl, pound bananas well with a fork or potato masher.
- Add vanilla, maple syrup, and coconut milk.
- Whisk everything together well, and afterward adds to dry ingredients. Blend until just mixed.
- Overlay in walnuts.
- A split blend between biscuit tins.
- Sprinkle biscuit tops with coconut.
- Prepare 23-27 minutes, or until tops simply start to firm and coconut starts to brown.

Chapter: 2 Lunch

18: Turmeric Tofu Scramble

Tofu can be scary, yet this flexible plant protein takes on whatever flavor you give it. With each chomp of this exquisite scramble recipe, you'll feel better and stimulated. This morning meal will likewise help deal with your glucose levels. This turmeric tofu scramble is made with delightful, supplement-pressed flavors and is an amazing plant-based option in contrast to your commonplace egg-driven lunch.

Ingredients:

- 1 teaspoon turmeric powder
- 2 tablespoons healthful yeast (optional)
- 1/4 teaspoon cayenne pepper
- freshly ground black pepper (MUST)
- 2 tablespoons non-dairy milk or Veganaise
- grapeseed oil for cooking
- 1/2 teaspoon fine ocean salt
- 1/2 bundle (15 oz.) natural firm tofu (grew is extraordinary as well)

Method:

- Channel the tofu from the water and break the tofu into little scraps.
- Add the nourishing yeast, turmeric, pepper, salt, and milk, and mix well.
- Heat nonstick skillet on a low heat, then add oil.
- Add the tofu into the skillet and cook for around 3-4 minutes mixing sporadically.
- Add the child spinach and cover with a top to permit the heat to steam the spinach.
- Turn the heat off when you do this and reveal and two or multiple times more.
- Serve hot with cherry tomatoes and avocado toast. (red peppers or different veggies likewise work incredibly, however, tomatoes are a lot speedier to cook and the concentration here is 5 minutes.

19: Shredded Brussels Sprouts with Bacon and Onions

Shredded Brussels sprouts are my #1 fresh dish, truly give me a fork. It's a side dish that meets up super-quick. Each chomp is stacked with flavor, toss with garlic, and finished off with a firm, smoky bacon. It makes the whole cycle a lot simpler and truly shreds the fledglings into a flawless knot of green. You can likewise utilize a sharp blade and get the cuts as slim as could be expected.

Ingredients:

- 4 cups chicken stock or low-sodium stock
- Coarse salt and freshly ground pepper
- 1 Spanish onion, daintily cut
- 8 garlic cloves, split the long way
- 4 pounds Brussels sprouts, managed
- 1/2 pound thickly cut lean bacon, cut across into flimsy strips
- Sugar (optional)

Method:

- In a big, profound skillet, cook the bacon over tolerably high heat until caramelized, around 8 minutes.
- Add the onion and garlic, reduce the heat to direct, and cook, mixing, until relaxed, around 5 minutes.
- Add the stock, season with salt and pepper and a spot of sugar, and cook until the fluid has reduced to 1 cup, around 12 minutes.
- Then, in a large pot of bubbling salted water, whiten the Brussels sprouts until scarcely delicate, around 3 minutes.
- Add the fledglings to the skillet. Stew delicately over moderate heat, mixing every so often, until delicate all through, around 10 minutes; season with salt and pepper.
- Utilizing an opened spoon, move to a bowl.

- Heat the fluid in the skillet over tolerably high heat until reduced to 1/2 cup. Pour the sauce over the Brussels fledglings and serve.

20: Vegan Coconut Kefir Banana Muffins

These biscuits taste natural and consoling, given their feathery, banana-mixed internal parts. They're also fun and tropical, because of the Shredded coconut you'll discover within and on the biscuit tops. A little lemon zing unites every one of the flavors.

These biscuits are improved with essentially ready bananas, with simply a trace of coconut palm sugar (or brown sugar). If you don't have these elective flours available, simply supplant them with wheat or gluten-free flour of your decision. With just 10 ingredients, these sound, plant-based biscuits are not difficult to heat up, and they will be a certain fire hit with the whole family.

Ingredients:

- ½ cup virgin coconut oil, dissolved
- ¼ cup honey
- 1 ½ teaspoon preparing powder
- ¼ teaspoon fine ocean salt
- ½ cup white whole wheat flour or ordinary whole wheat flour
- ¾ cup unsweetened Shredded coconut, isolated
- 1 tablespoon turbinado (crude) sugar
- ½ teaspoon lemon zing (the zing from about ½ medium lemon)
- 1 cup squashed ready banana (from around 3 bananas)
- 1 big egg, ideally at room temperature
- 1 teaspoon vanilla concentrate

- ¾ cup whole wheat baked good flour or white/standard whole wheat flour

Method:

- Preheat stove to 375 degrees Fahrenheit. If important, oil every one of the 12 cups of your biscuit tin with spread or biscuit liners (my dish is non-stick and didn't need any oil).
- In a medium bowl, whisk together the flours, salt, heating powder, and lemon zing. Mix in ½ cup of the shredded coconut.
- In a different, medium bowl, whisk together the pounded banana, honey, coconut oil, egg, and vanilla.
- Empty the wet ingredients into the dry ingredients and mix until just consolidated.
- Separation the player uniformly between the biscuit cups (a meager ¼ cup hitter every), then sprinkle the biscuit tops with the excess ¼ cup Shredded coconut.
- Sprinkle the tops with crude sugar.
- Prepare for around 17 to 20 minutes, until a toothpick embedded into the middle, tells the truth.
- Move biscuits to a cooling rack and let them cool.

21: Avocado Ricotta Power Toast

This avocado toast gets a novel turn with extra garnishes of lemon ricotta, kale microgreens, and a sprinkle of all that bagel zest. This ricotta avocado toast is uncommonly acceptable, getting its splendid, fresh taste from the lemony ricotta. The pillowy ricotta shapes the base for the avocado which gets finished off with a runny egg for additional flavor. Polished off with a sprinkling of fragile microgreens and a sprinkle of all that bagel zest, this toast shines a different light on the words simple, workday breakfast.

Ingredients:

- 4 eggs
- 6 tablespoons ricotta cheddar
- 3 avocados, crushed
- 4 tablespoons harissa
- 4 cups of whole wheat, toasted
- 1/4 cup cut green onions
- 1 teaspoon white vinegar

Method:

- Fill a big skillet around 1/2″ loaded with water.
- Heat to the point of boiling.
- Add bread to toaster oven and toast until somewhat sautéed.
- Eliminate and let sit.
- Add a sprinkle of white vinegar to the bubbling water (around 1 teaspoon).
- Quickly include 4 eggs separating them. Cover.
- Turn burners off.
- Leave eggs covered with the heat off for 4-5 minutes.
- Meanwhile, add 1/2 tablespoons of ricotta to each piece of toast, just as 1/4 cup of squashed avocado, and 1 tablespoon of harissa.
- When eggs poached.
- Delicately eliminate from water (make certain to empty any fluid of the skillet) and spot on top of amassed toast.
- Embellishment with green onions.
- Serve!

22: Vegan Lentil Burgers

Burgers will consistently be one of my #1 food varieties! These Completely Vegan Lentil Burgers permit you to appreciate this exemplary fave yet in a MUCH better manner! Every burger contains such a lot of plant-based goodness; your body will much be obliged.

These fiery Vegan Lentil Burgers are made with split red lentils and are finished off with the most delectable rich vegetarian avocado sauce. Prepared in less than 20 minutes, these lentil patties are extraordinary as burgers, lettuce wraps, or in a salad.

Ingredients:

- 1 onion, slashed
- ½ pound (227 g) of mushrooms, freshly cut
- 2 tablespoons (30 mL) of vegetable oil
- 2 cups (500 mL) of cooked lentils
- 4 cloves of garlic, freshly slashed
- 1 cup (250 mL) of bread morsels
- 2 tablespoons (30 mL) of dried thyme
- ½ cup (125 mL) of nut or almond margarine
- ¼ cup (60 mL) of chia seeds
- 2 tablespoons (30 mL) of miso glue
- 2 tablespoons (30 mL) of soy sauce
- 2 cups (500 mL) of yam, ground

Method:

- Sprinkle the oil into your skillet over medium-high heat.

- Toss in the mushrooms, onion, and garlic, and sauté until they become brown and tasty around 10 minutes. Move the mix to your food processor.
- Add every one of the excess ingredients except the ground yam. Puree the combination until everything is easily joined.
- Move the combination to a mixing bowl and mix in the yam by hand so it doesn't separate in the machine.
- Rest the combination for ten minutes, giving the chia seeds time to do something amazing.
- Utilizing your hands, shape the mix into equally framed patties.
- They might be cooked promptly, refrigerated for a few days, or frozen for a month.
- When the time has come to cook you have heaps of alternatives for these burgers.
- You may broil them in a daintily oiled sauté skillet on your burner, singe them on your iron, barbecue, or BBQ, or even prepare in your broiler at 400°F (200°C) for 15 to 20 minutes.
- Whatever method you pick, remember that these burgers brown moderately rapidly so medium-high heat will permit the focuses to keep up while the outsides cook.

23: Baked Mahi Mahi

It's an incredible, more affordable option in contrast to halibut, and can be barbecued, cooked, or even singed. Yet, one of our number one different ways to set it up is to just dish burn it, which lets the flavors and flaky surface sparkle. Singing it in a skillet also allows you to make a rich, lemony sauce to shower everywhere on the fish. All you need to finish this simple fish meal is a green salad or vegetable, and possibly some bread or rice to sop up all that delectable sauce. Here's the simplest method to cook mahi mahi.

Ingredients:

- ¼ tsp salt
- ¾ cup cream
- ¼ tsp pepper
- ½ cup raspberry juice
- ¼ cup balsamic vinegar
- 1 tbsp. spread
- 6-piece medium size mahi-mahi

Method:

- Spread 1 tablespoon of margarine on 6 bits of medium-sized mahi-mahi and sprinkle it with 1/4 teaspoon every one of pepper and salt.
- Orchestrate the fishes on a lubed heating dish. Pour 3/4 cup of cream and 1/4 cup of Balsamic vinegar over the fish.
- Cover the heating dish with material paper and spot it inside a broiler that has been preheated to 450 degrees Fahrenheit. Cook for 12 minutes.

24: Grass-Fed Burgers

If you've changed to grass-took care of meat, you likely realize that it's liberated from chemicals and lower in fat, and higher in some significant supplements than ordinary grain-took care of hamburger. If you bought it simply from a limited-scale farmer, you may likewise be aware of subtleties like the cows' variety and age.

Ingredients:

- 4 teaspoons fit salt
- 2 lbs. Belcampo ground hamburger
- 4 Slices provolone cheddar
- 8 Slices cooked bacon
- 4 Brioche burger buns
- 4 Slices tomato and other burger garnishes (pickles, red onion)

Method:

- Separation 2 lbs. grass-took care of hamburger into four segments.
- To not exhaust the meat, eliminate it from the bundle and simply shape it into burger patties around 5" across – don't massage the meat.
- Sprinkle every burger with one teaspoon Kosher salt partitioned one half on each side
- Preheat barbecue on high
- Cook for 3 minutes on each side for Medium Rare, 4 minutes on each side for Medium. Eliminate from heat when inner temp arrives at 125F.
- Spot cheddar on the burger after the main flip
- Eliminate from the flame broil and spot on a bun with garnish and cooked Bacon

25: Cinnamon Roll Fat Bombs

The cinnamon fat bombs are made keto-accommodating by keeping the ingredients low carb and high fat, and the cream cheddar icing is amazingly acceptable. This is genuinely a high-fat keto bite that is amazing. Here's a recipe for making cinnamon simply move fat bombs.

Ingredients:

- ½ cup almond flour
- ½ cup unsalted margarine, at room temperature
- 1 tsp ground cinnamon
- 3 ½ tbsp. granulated Stevia or another granulated sugar to taste
- For cream cheddar icing:
- ½ tsp vanilla concentrate
- 3 tbsp. cream cheddar
- 1 ½ tbsp. substantial cream
- 1 ½ tbsp. granulated Stevia or another granulated low carb sugar to taste

Method:

- In a bowl place the spread and granulated Stevia and utilizing an electric mixer beat on medium speed until mixed.
- Add the almond flour and cinnamon and beat to consolidate.
- Cover the batter and refrigerate for 30 minutes or until adequately hard to frame balls.
- Free the mixture once again from the fridge and fold into balls around 1 tablespoon in size.
- Freeze the balls for 20 minutes.
- To make the icing, in a microwave-safe bowl join every one of the ingredients.
- Microwave on high for 20 seconds.
- Eliminate from the microwave and mix.
- Shower the icing over the balls.
- Keep the balls in a water/airproof holder in the fridge until prepared to serve.

26: Cauliflower Popcorn

This low-carb cauliflower popcorn is perhaps the yummiest (and generally fun!) approach to eat cauliflower. No spongy business here! With its wonderfully firm covering, this dish is a hit with the whole family, if they are watching their carbs. Functions admirably as finger food, as an hors d'oeuvre, or as a side dish.

Ingredients:

- 1 cup (75g) panko breadcrumbs
- 1 teaspoon smoked paprika

- 1 Coles Australian Free Range Egg, delicately whisked
- 2 teaspoons coarsely chopped thyme twigs
- 1 cauliflower, cut into little florets
- 1/2 cup (40g) finely ground parmesan

Method:

- Preheat stove to 200°C. Line a preparing plate with heating paper.
- Cook the cauliflower in a big pot of bubbling water for 5 mins or until simply delicate. Channel well.
- Move to a big bowl. Mix in the egg.
- Consolidate the breadcrumbs, parmesan, paprika, and thyme in a big bowl. Add the cauliflower mix and toss to join.
- Mastermind the mix in a solitary layer over the lined plate. Shower well with olive oil splash. Season.

27: Best Baked Potato

This heated potato recipe is pretty much as a clear record as it gets. Don't hesitate to add different flavors to the salt-and-pepper mix, like cumin or smoked paprika, and get done with whatever cheddar you like. In case you're utilizing little potatoes, you can slice them down the middle or if they're minuscule, you can simply give them a little jab with a fork or blade before preparing to permit the steam to getaway.

Ingredients:

- 1/4 cup olive oil
- 1 tablespoon salt
- 4 big Russet potatoes

Method:

- Preheat the stove to 425 degrees.
- Wash and dry the potatoes.
- Puncture the potato 2-3 times with a fork
- Rub oil everywhere on the potatoes (or pick one of the different alternatives above to rub outwardly).
- Rub salt everywhere on the potatoes. We incline toward coarse ocean salt or pink Himalayan salt.
- Spot the potatoes on a preparing sheet and heat for around 45 minutes.
- The specific preparing time will rely upon how big the potatoes are. The potato ought to be delicate inside if you stick a fork into it.
- Present with spread, chives, cheddar, sharp cream, and the entirety of your #1 garnishes!

28: Crispy Cauliflower Pizza Crust

Cauliflower Pizza Crust is extremely popular however if you don't make it effectively, it tends to be a spongy disillusionment. The objective is to have a decent firm hull, not a limp, soft wreck. After much experimentation, we at last sorted out the key to the whole fresh Cauliflower Pizza Crust.

This cauliflower pizza outside layer recipe utilizes basic ingredients with the goal that you can the entirety of the tasty garnishes you like. It's low carb, gluten-free, without grain, and pressing the flavor. This is what you'll have to make it:

Ingredients:

- 2 pounds' cauliflower florets riced
- 1 egg beaten
- 1 teaspoon dried oregano
- 1/4 teaspoon Himalayan salt

- 1/2 cup ground mozzarella cheddar or Parmesan cheddar

Method:

- Preheat stove to 400 degrees F.
- Heartbeat bunches of crude cauliflower florets in a food processor, until a rice-like surface, is accomplished. However, don't over-cycle or cream it.
- Microwave the cauliflower rice for around 1 moment or until delicate. Or heat it: In a large pot, load up with about an inch of water, and heat it to the point of boiling.
- Add the cauliflower "rice" and cover. Cook around 4-5 minutes. After the cauliflower is cooked, channel it into a fine sifter or over cheesecloth.
- On your counter over a towel, spread out a fine-network cheesecloth.
- Pour the mix on the cheesecloth and utilizing the cheesecloth, assemble and press out any additional dampness into the sink.
- Pat much more dampness out by tapping again with the towel. Ensure all the water is taken out by crushing out on the towel.
- Whenever dampness is taken out, move "rice" to a large mixing bowl. Add beaten egg, cheddar, oregano, and salt. You may have to utilize your hands to mix.
- Press the mixture out onto a heating sheet fixed with material paper.
- Utilizing hands press level and crush in the sides to frame a shape at ⅓ inch high. Make marginally higher on the sides.

- Heat 35-40 minutes at 400 degrees F or until the outside layer is firm and amazing brown.
- Eliminate from broiler and add garnishes.
- Heat an extra 5-10 minutes until cheddar is hot and effervescent. Serve right away.

29: Almond Apple Spice Muffins

These paleo apple biscuits are so fast and simple to assemble thus great! Heat them toward the end of the week and freeze for in and out morning meals during the week. They're gluten-free and without grain with a sans dairy alternative.

Ingredients:

- 1 teaspoon allspice
- 1 teaspoon cloves
- 2 cups almond meal
- 4 eggs
- 1 cup unsweetened fruit purée
- 5 scoops of vanilla protein powder
- 1/2 stick margarine
- 1 tablespoon cinnamon

Method:

- Preheat the broiler to 350 degrees. Liquefy margarine in the microwave (~30 seconds on low heat).
- Completely mix every one of the ingredients in a bowl.
- Splash biscuit tin with non-stick cooking shower or use cupcake liners.
- Empty mix into biscuit tins, make a point, not to overload (~3/4 full); this should make 12 biscuits (2 biscuit plate).
- Spot one plate in the broiler and cook for 12 minutes.

- Make a point not to overcook as the biscuits will turn out to be extremely dry.
- When cooked, eliminate from the broiler and cook the second biscuit plate.

30: Healthy Mexican Fried Rice

This Mexican singed rice recipe is also an extraordinary method to rapidly make a side dish utilizing precooked rice from a clump cooking meeting or extra rice. The way to making incredible singed rice is utilizing cooked, cold rice. When I make any kind of singed rice recipe, I like to clump cook rice the other day and refrigerate it short-term so it gets quite cold. Cooked rice also freezes well if you needed to make a bigger group and freeze it in the sums you need for this and other rice plans.

Ingredients:

- 2 teaspoons olive oil
- 100 grams (1/2 cup) brown rice
- 1 little yellow onion, sliced
- 1 garlic clove, squashed
- 1 little bean stew pepper, deseeded and chopped
- 1 teaspoon Mexican stew powder
- 1/2 can corn portions
- 1/2 can black beans, washed
- 1 tablespoon fresh lime juice
- 100-gram grape tomatoes, chopped
- Fresh coriander, to serve
- Lime wedges, to serve
- 60-gram feta disintegrated
- 1/4 little red onion, finely slashed
- 1/2 little avocado, quartered and cut

Method:

- Cook the rice in a large pan of bubbling water for 25 minutes or until delicate.
- Channel well, then spread onto a large plate and spot into the ice chest, uncovered, for at any rate 60 minutes.
- Heat the oil in a big griddle over medium heat.
- Add the yellow onion and stew pepper, and cook for five minutes or until delicate. Add the garlic and bean stew powder.
- Proceed to cook and mix for 30 seconds or until fragrant.
- Add the rice and cook, mixing, for two minutes until softly seared and all around joined with the onion mix.
- Add the beans and corn and keep cooking, mixing regularly, until warmed through. Pour lime squeeze over and toss to consolidate.
- Consolidate the tomatoes and red onion and season to taste.
- Split the rice mix between serving bowls and top with the tomato combination, feta, avocado, coriander, and lime wedges.

31: Turkey Tacos

Here is another best recipe for your lunch. This recipe has a couple of stunts at its disposal to ensure each chomp is delicious and completely prepared. Coming to tortillas close to you in around 15 minutes.

Ingredients:

- 8 taco shells
- 1 tablespoon olive oil

- 1-pound ground turkey
- 1 little yellow onion, slashed
- ½ teaspoon bean stew powder
- Salt
- 1 ½ cups (6 ounces) shredded Cheddar
- 1 little head of romaine lettuce, Shredded
- 1 beefsteak tomato, cubed

Method:

- Heat the oil in a medium heat.
- Add the onion and cook, mixing, until marginally delicate, around 4 minutes.
- Add the turkey and cook, disintegrating with the rear of a spoon, until no hint of pink remaining parts, 5 to 7 minutes.
- Mix in the bean stew powder and ½ teaspoon salt.
- Spoon the filling into the taco shells and top with lettuce, Cheddar, and tomato.

32: Healthy Spaghetti Bolognese

Making hand-crafted bolognese sauce is simpler than you'd suspect! This healthy bolognese is a delectable, flavorful dish that you can make without any preparation in just 25 minutes.

Ingredients:

- 2 garlic cloves, stripped and finely sliced
- 1 tsp light olive oil
- 1 medium onion, finely sliced
- 1 medium courgette, finely cubed
- 1 celery sticks, finely sliced
- 600ml meat stock
- 400g turkey mince

- 1 big carrot, ground
- 2 sound leaves
- 300g whole-wheat spaghetti
- 150ml red wine (optional)
- 400g tin sliced tomatoes
- Parmesan shavings, to serve
- basil leaves, to serve

Method:

- Heat the oil in a big, non-stick, weighty lined pan.
- Add the onion, celery, and 2 tablespoons water and fry for 5 minutes or until the vegetables have mellowed.
- Add the courgette and fry for another 2-3 minutes.
- Add the mince and garlic and fry for another 3-4 minutes, mixing now and again or until the mince has separated and is beginning to brown. Mix well.
- Add the ground carrot and 150ml of the hamburger stock or red wine, whenever liked, and stew for 3-4 minutes.
- Then add the tinned tomatoes, 450ml hamburger stock, and the narrows leaves and bring them to the heat.
- Cover with a top, turn down the heat to medium-low, and leave to stew for 45 minutes, mixing once in a while.
- Eliminate the cover and cook for another 10-15 minutes, or until the fluid has reduced and thickened to wanted consistency.
- Cook the spaghetti as per parcel directions, channel, and split between 6 plates. Spot a spoonful of Bolognese on top of each plate, dissipate with basil leaves and Parmesan shavings.

The trail mix nibble recipe I am showing you today is exceptionally healthy since it is wealthy in cancer prevention agents. As you may know, cell reinforcements advance great wellbeing as they help stay away from infections. All the more explicitly, cancer prevention agents help hinder the oxidation of cells in our body.

When cells oxidize, they create free extremists, which are otherwise called cell bi-items. It is protected to have a sensible measure of these free revolutionaries in the body. Notwithstanding, when the free revolutionaries are in abundance, they can unleash ruin on our organic entity's cell mechanical assembly.

Ingredients:

- Cheerios
- Wheat, corn, or rice Chex cereal
- Low-fat popcorn
- Low-fat granola cereal bunches
- Low-fat sesame seeds
- Unsalted pretzel winds or sticks
- Unsalted sunflower seeds (shelled)
- Sans sugar chocolate chips or M&Ms
- Soy nuts
- Unsalted scaled-down rice cakes

Method:

- You can likewise buy low sugar or sans sugar dried fruit at different wellbeing food stores.
- Likewise, one of the most reduced sugar-dried fruits is apple.

- Figs are another healthy decision.
- If you should utilize high glossed-over treats, use them with some restraint.
- While setting up these treats, you can toss them in close Ziploc baggies that are not difficult to bring on picnics, strolls, or any place you go.

34: Weight Watchers Berry Crisp

This Weight Watchers Berry Crisp is a delightful and simple sweet you don't need to feel remorseful about enjoying. This fast, 5-ingredient treat hits every one of the spots of those old top choices yet with way fewer calories. The recipe is made with fresh berries and improved with a dash of brown sugar and a trace of cinnamon. It's done off with a fresh ingredient made of low-fat granola.

Ingredients:

- 1½ cups raspberries
- 1½ cups fresh blackberries
- 1½ cups blueberries
- ¾ cup generally useful flour
- ¼ cup sugar
- ½ cup amazing brown sugar, stuffed
- ¾ cup moved oats
- ½ teaspoon cinnamon
- Fat-free frozen vanilla yogurt, optional
- ½ cup reduced-fat margarine, cold
- Gently whipped cream, optional

Method:

- Preheat broiler to 350 degrees

- In a medium bowl utilizing an elastic spatula, delicately toss together the blackberries, raspberries, blueberries, and white sugar; put in a safe spot
- In a different medium bowl, join flour, oats, brown sugar, and cinnamon. Add the margarine in pieces and cautiously mix while keeping brittle.
- Coat 6 (3 ½-inch) ramekins with a cooking splash, see prep tip. Split the sugared berries between them.
- Separation and sprinkle equitably absurd the disintegrate mix, about ⅓ cup for each.
- Line a preparing sheet with material paper or foil. Spot the 6 ramekin cups on the skillet.
- Prepare for around 40 minutes until amazing brown. Top with a little whipped cream or frozen yogurt, whenever wanted.

35: San Choy Bau Bowl

San Choy Bau is one of those dishes my children continue to request over and over. It's an incredible one for outdoors in the light of the fact that the ingredients store effectively (clam sauce ought to be kept in the refrigerator), and you just need one skillet. A similar sum functions as a starter for a large gathering (diamond lettuce goes home better for this) – or feed the family as a simple without carb lunch.

Ingredients:

- 500g pork mince
- 1 tablespoon ground ginger
- 1/4 cup clam sauce
- 2 garlic cloves, finely slashed
- 1 tablespoon nut oil
- 2 tablespoons kecap manis

- 2 teaspoons lime juice
- 1/2 tablespoon caster sugar
- 1 teaspoon sesame oil
- coriander leaves
- 1 little chunk of ice lettuce
- salted carrots
- singed shallots
- 1/4 cup slashed peanuts, gently cooked with salt

Method:

- Heat the nut oil in a wok over high heat.
- Add the pork mince, garlic, and ginger to the wok and cook through. Channel off any fluid to guarantee the mince is very dry.
- In a little bowl join the shellfish sauce, caster sugar, kecap manis, lime juice, and sesame oil.
- Add 66% of the sauce to the pork mince and mix through a few minutes until the sauce thickens.
- Eliminate the wok from the heat and permit the mince to cool marginally.
- In a little, dry fry container, toast the peanuts and put them to the side to cool.
- Wash, dry, and trim your lettuce leaves and spread them out on a plate.
- Split the mince combination between the lettuce cups.
- Top each San Choy Bau with salted carrot, broiled peanuts, coriander leaves, and seared shallots.
- Spoon over the leftover sauce.

36: Sheet Pan Steak

To make a sheet dish form of this exemplary meal, broil the potatoes until delicate and afterward cook everything under the oven to give it an amazing brown burn. Sheet Pan Steak and Potatoes conveys all the generous solace however practically no dishes to tidy up.

Ingredients:

- 1 head of broccoli, cut into florets
- 1/4 cup olive oil
- 2 tablespoons fresh rosemary, minced (or 2 teaspoons dry, squashed)
- 2 tablespoons balsamic vinegar
- Fit salt
- 9 cloves garlic, minced and isolated
- Fresh broke black pepper
- 1/2 pounds Yukon gold potatoes, split
- 2 pounds of level iron steak (can substitute flank steak simply try to check the inward temp)

Method:

- Preheat broiler to 450°. Line a large rimmed heating sheet with foil.
- Spot the steak in a large zipper-top pack with the 1/4 cup olive oil, 4 cloves of garlic, salt, vinegar, balsamic and pepper.
- Go to cover and let marinate at any rate 1 hour as long as 8 hours.
- Disperse potatoes and rosemary on the heating sheet and shower with 1 tablespoon of olive oil, and season with salt and pepper.
- Toss tenderly with utensils to cover and spread them out equitably.
- Cook potatoes mix until they start to brown around the edges, around 20 minutes.

- Join the leftover 2 tablespoons of olive oil, broccoli, and remaining garlic in a bowl; season with salt and pepper, and toss to cover. Spot on the heating sheet alongside the potatoes.
- Spot an ovenproof wire rack over the broccoli and potatoes. Eliminate the steak from the zip-top sack and shake off the abundance marinade. Lay the steak on the rack.
- Return the preparing sheet to the broiler and dish until a moment read thermometer embedded evenly into the focal point of meat registers 125, around 10 to 15 minutes.
- Eliminate from the broiler and let rest for 5 to 10 minutes before cutting.

37: Poached Eggs and Avocado Toasts

Make the most of your day away from work with a nutritious and healthy lunch with this Avocado Toast with Poached Egg. A basic simple avocado concoction spread on a cut of toasted wholegrain bread and finished off with a poached egg. It is flavorful. This fair may turn into a customary thing on your lunch menu.

You need a wonderfully ready avocado and a pleasant thick cut of fresh bread to toast. Since avocados become brown when the fruit is presented to the air, pound it up with a little lemon squeeze then sprinkle some salt in to draw out the flavor.

Ingredients:

- 2 eggs
- salt and pepper for ingredient
- 2 cups of wholegrain bread

- 2 tablespoons shaved Parmesan cheddar
- quartered treasure tomatoes for serving
- fresh spices (parsley, thyme, or basil) for ingredient
- 1/3 avocado (for the most part I cut it down the middle yet don't utilize every last bit of it. alright fine perhaps I do.)

Method:

- Carry a pot of water to heat (utilize sufficient water to cover the eggs when they lay in the base).
- Drop the metal edges (external edge just) of two artisan container covers into the pot so they are laying level on the base.
- When the water is bubbling, turn off the heat and cautiously break the eggs simply into each edge.
- Cover the pot and poach for 5 minutes (4 for too delicate, 4:30 for delicate, at least 5 for semi-delicate yolks).
- While the eggs are cooking, toast the bread and crush the avocado on each piece of toast.
- When the eggs are done, utilize a spatula to lift the eggs out of the water. Delicately remove the edge from the eggs (I do this privilege on the spatula, over the water) and spot the poached eggs on top of the toast.
- Sprinkle with Parmesan cheddar, salt, pepper, and fresh spices; present with the fresh quartered legacy tomatoes.

38: Veggie-Packed Cheesy Chicken Salad

These veggie-pressed dinners will have you covered from breakfast to dinner. Furthermore, these plans have close to 15 grams of sugars for every serving. Plans like Green Shakshuka and Buffalo Chicken Cauliflower Pizza are vivid, scrumptious, and brimming with supplements and nutrients.

Ingredients:

- 1 lb. uncooked slight cut chicken breasts
- 7 tablespoons diminished fat balsamic vinaigrette dressing
- 1 medium zucchini (8 oz.), cut the long way down the middle
- 1 medium red onion, cut into 1/4-inch cuts
- 4 plum (Roma) tomatoes, cut down the middle
- 6 cups torn arugula
- ½ cup disintegrated feta cheddar (2 oz.)

Method:

- Heat gas or charcoal barbecue. Brush chicken with 1 tablespoon of the dressing. Cautiously brush oil on the barbecue rack.
- Spot chicken, zucchini, and onion on flame broil over medium heat.
- Cover flame broil; cook 8 to 10 minutes, turning once, until chicken is not, at this point pink in focus and vegetables are delicate.
- Add tomato parts to flame broil throughout the previous 4 minutes of cooking.

- Reduce chicken and vegetables from flame broil to cutting board.
- Cut chicken across into slender cuts; coarsely cleave vegetables.
- In a large bowl, throw chicken, vegetables, and the leftover 6 tablespoons of dressing.
- Add arugula and cheddar; throw tenderly. Serve right away.

39: Cobb Salad with Brown Derby Dressing

The recipe contained in this Cobb Salad with French Dressing was given to me by Walt Disney World Guest Services or a Disney Chef at the eatery. The recipe in Cobb Salad with French Dressing may have been downsized by the Disney Chefs for the home culinary specialist. We love this salad. It's expensive even by Disney principles yet it genuinely is scrumptious.

Salad ingredients:

- 1/2 package watercress
- 3 eggs, hard-cooked
- 1/2 head icy mass lettuce
- 1 little pack chicory
- 2 medium tomatoes, whitened and stripped
- 1/2 head romaine lettuce
- 1/2 cups cooked turkey breast, cubed
- 2 tablespoons slashed chives
- 6 strips fresh bacon, disintegrated
- 1/2 cup blue cheddar, disintegrated

French Dressing Ingredients:

- 1/2 teaspoon sugar

- 1/2 cup water
- 1/4 tablespoons salt
- 1 clove garlic, chopped
- 1/2 cups salad oil
- 1/2 cup red wine vinegar
- 1/2 teaspoons Worcestershire sauce
- Juice of 1/2 lemon
- 1/2 teaspoon English mustard
- 1/2 cup olive oil
- 1/2 tablespoon ground dark pepper

Method for Cobb Salad:

- Slash all greens fine and mastermind in a salad bowl.
- Cut tomatoes down the middle, reduce seeds, and dice fine.
- Likewise dice the turkey, avocado, and eggs.
- Mastermind the above ingredients, just as the blue cheddar and bacon disintegrate, in straight lines across the greens.
- Mastermind the chives slantingly across the above lines.
- Present the salad at the table, then throw it with the dressing.
- Spot on chilled plates with a watercress enhancement.

Method for Dressing:

- Mix all ingredients aside from oils.
- Then add olive oil and salad oils and blend well.
- Mix well again before blending in with the salad.

Thai Noodle Salad with the BEST EVER Peanut Sauce- stacked up with sound veggies! This veggie lover salad is incredible for potlucks and Sunday dinner - prep and keeps going as long as 5 days in the refrigerator. Gluten-free versatile. Incorporates a 35-second video.

Ingredients:

- 4 cups blend of cabbage, carrots, and radish, destroyed or ground
- 6-ounce dry noodles (earthy colored rice noodles, cushion Thai style rice noodles, soba noodles, linguini)
- 3 scallions, cut
- 1 red chime pepper, finely cut
- ½ pack cilantro, chopped (or sub basil and mint)
- ¼–½ cup broiled, squashed peanuts (embellish)
- 1 tablespoon jalapeño (finely chopped)

Method:

- Cook pasta as per bearings on the package.
- Channel and chill under cool running water.
- Throw: Place destroyed veggies, chime pepper, scallions, cilantro, and jalapeño into a serving bowl. Throw.
- Add the chilly noodles to the serving bowl and throw once more. Pour the nut sauce up and over and throw well to join.
- (However you would prefer), add stew drops if you need and serve, decorating with broiled peanuts and cilantro and a lime wedge.

If you're in the disposition for a dinner salad that is generous, solid, and heavenly, then look no farther than this Roasted Vegetable and Farro Salad. This salad joins nutty, chewy faro with an assortment of broiled vegetables, all threw in a balsamic vinaigrette and present with disintegrated feta.

Ingredients:

- ⅔ cup broccoli florets
- 1½ cups cooked farro
- ¼ cup grape tomatoes divided
- ½ of ringer pepper, chopped
- ¼ of zucchini, cubed
- 1 tsp olive oil
- 1 tsp ocean salt + more to taste
- 1 clove garlic, shredded
- 1 tsp dried or fresh rosemary
- 4-5 kalamata olives, cut
- 2 tbsp. disintegrated goat cheddar
- ¼ cup pecan parts, slashed

Method:

- Preheat the broiler to 400°F and fix a skillet with material paper.
- Throw broccoli, tomatoes, zucchini, and ringer pepper with olive oil, rosemary, salt, and shredded garlic in a bowl until equally covered.
- Spread on arranged dish and meal in preheated broiler for 25 minutes.
- Joined broiled vegetables with cooked farro, cut olives, and pecans.

- Add salt to taste.
- Top with disintegrated goat cheddar and serve.

42: Cajun Potato, Shrimp, and Avocado Salad

We have another best recipe in our book that is Cajun Potato, Shrimp, and Avocado Salad. It is the best discontinuous fasting recipe to attempt. Many people like it and it is not difficult to make.

Ingredients:

- 2 spring onions (finely cut)
- 2 teaspoons Cajun preparing
- 1 garlic clove (shredded)
- 1 tablespoon oil (olive oil)
- 1 avocado (stripped, stoned, and cubed)
- 1 cup horse feed sprout
- Salt (to bubble potatoes)
- 300-gram potatoes (fresh potatoes, little child or talks 10 oz. divided)
- 250-gram crude shrimp (ruler prawns, 8 oz., cooked and stripped)

Method:

- Cook the potatoes in an enormous pot of delicately salted bubbling water for 10 to 15 minutes or until delicate, channel well.
- Heat the oil in a wok or large nonstick griddle/skillet.
- Add the prawns, garlic, spring onions, and Cajun preparing and pan sear for 2 to 3 minutes or until the prawns are hot.
- Mix in the potatoes and cook briefly.

- Move to serve dishes and top with the avocado and the hay fledglings and serve.

43: Simple Black Bean Soup

It is a basic and solid soup made with canned dark beans and regular ingredients! This delightful dark bean soup is veggie-lover, without gluten, and vegan. This soup is ideal for lunch, occupied weeknights, or taking care of an eager group. Our whole family cherishes this soup and we as a whole get energized when it's on the menu! It hits the recognize without fail.

Ingredients:

- 1 medium red onion, finely chopped
- 2 tbsp. extra-virgin olive oil
- 2 cloves garlic, shredded
- 1 tbsp. tomato glue
- 1 tbsp. shredded jalapeños
- salt
- 1 tsp. bean stew powder
- Freshly ground dark pepper
- 1/2 tsp. cumin
- 3 (15-oz.) jars dark beans, with fluid
- 1 bay leaf
- 1 qt. low-sodium chicken or vegetable stock
- acrid cream, for embellish
- Cleaved fresh cilantro, for embellish
- Cut avocado, to decorate

Method:

- In an enormous pot over medium heat, heat oil. Add onion and cook until delicate and clear, around 5 minutes.
- Add jalapeños and garlic and cook until fragrant, around 2 minutes.
- Add tomato glue, mix to cover vegetables, and cook about a brief more. Season with salt, bean stew powder, pepper, and cumin and mix to cover.
- Add dark beans with their fluid and chicken stock. Mix soup, add cove leaf and heat to the point of boiling.
- Quickly decrease to a stew and let stew until marginally diminished around 15 minutes. Reduce inlet leaf.
- Utilizing a drenching blender or food processor, mix the soup to wanted consistency.
- Present with a touch of sharp cream, cut avocado, and cilantro.

44: Chicken with Fried Cauliflower Rice

This Chicken Fried Cauliflower Rice is not difficult to make and can be filled in as your principal dish or as a side dish. It's low in focuses, low in carbs, and loaded up with veggies and protein. It is a fast and simple Asian one container supper recipe that the whole family will cherish.

Ingredients:

- 2 big eggs
- 1 tablespoon sesame oil
- 1/2 cup chopped onion
- 2 tablespoons olive or avocado oil
- 1 clove garlic, crushed
- 1 teaspoon fresh ginger, crushed
- 4 teaspoons soy sauce, separated
- 1 cup cooked chicken
- 1 pound riced cauliflower
- 1/2 cup chopped scallions
- 1 tablespoon stew glue

Method:

- Heat oil in a big oven or wok over medium heat.
- Add the onion and cook, mixing regularly, until clear.
- Add the ginger, garlic, and chicken to the container and keep cooking for 2 minutes.
- Add the cauliflower to the oven and sprinkle with 3 teaspoons (1 tablespoon) of soy sauce and stew glue.

- Mix well and cook for 3 minutes or until the cauliflower has mollified.
- Push the cauliflower rice to the side of the dish and break the eggs into the unfilled space in the container. Sprinkle with 1 teaspoon soy sauce and scramble.
- When eggs are cooked through, mix the eggs into the rice.
- Remove from the heat and stir in the scallions.
- Sprinkle with sesame oil and serve.

45: Wild Cajun Spiced Salmon

Cajun Salmon with a simple natively constructed preparation made with flavors you as of now have in your washroom that can be heated, cooked, dish singed, or barbecued. This solid supper is prepared in under fifteen minutes and comparable to any eatery variant.

Cajun Salmon that is hot, smoky, and prepared right away makes for a simple and solid supper that can be cooked inside or outside on the flame broil. Serve it warm or cold for a protein-stuffed supper that is scrumptious. We likewise make this Blackened Salmon and Brown Sugar Salmon consistently, so add these to your go-to salmon plans.

Ingredients:

- 3 tsp olive oil, separated
- 2 6 oz. filets of salmon
- 2 tbsp. Cajun preparing
- Legitimate salt + broke black pepper, to taste

Method:

- Preheat the stove to 425 degrees C.
- Brush a preparing dish or oven with 1 tsp olive oil.

- Put salmon filets down into dish — skin-side down if they have skin.
- Brush 1 tsp of olive oil over each filet.
- Sprinkle with Kosher salt + broke black pepper.
- Sprinkle each filet with 1 tbsp. of Cajun preparing each, tapping and kneading the flavoring into the filet like a rub.
- Rub onto the sides of the filets too.
- Spot in the broiler and heat for 15 minutes or until filets effectively drop.
- The safe inward temperature for fish is 62.8 °C/145 °F.

46: Healthy Beef Stroganoff

This Healthy Beef Stroganoff recipe is outstanding both for what it offers—all the smooth, comfortable kind of the exemplary recipe, eased up with a couple of solid ingredient trades and made simpler in the simmering pot—just as for what it doesn't. This stewing pot meat stroganoff is made without canned soup.

Ingredients:

- 1 tablespoon margarine
- ½ teaspoon salt
- 1 teaspoon arranged mustard
- 2-pound meat hurl cook
- ½ teaspoon ground black pepper
- salt and ground black pepper to taste
- ⅓ cup white wine
- ¼ cup generally useful flour
- ½ pound white mushrooms, cut
- 1 ¼ cups decreased sodium meat stock, separated
- ⅓ cup light acrid cream

- 4 green onions, cut (white and green parts)
- 2 tablespoons spread, partitioned

Method:

- Remove any fat and cartilage from the meal and cut into strips 1/2-inch thick by 2-inches in length.
- Sprinkle with 1/2 teaspoon salt and 1/2 teaspoon pepper.
- Soften 1 tablespoon margarine in a large oven over medium heat.
- Add mushrooms and green onions and cook, mixing once in a while, until mushrooms are sautéed, around 6 minutes.
- Remove to a bowl and add 1 tablespoon margarine to the oven.
- Cook and mix one a large portion of the hamburger strips until caramelized, around 5 minutes, then remove to a bowl.
- Rehash with the excess spread and hamburger strips.
- Empty wine into the hot oven and deglaze the container, scraping up any sautéed bits.
- Join flour and 1/4 cup meat stock in a container with a firmly fitting cover and shake until consolidated.
- Stir into the oven, racing until smooth.
- Stir in the excess stock and mustard, then return the meat to the container.
- Bring to a stew. Cover and stew until the meat are delicate, around 60 minutes.
- Stir in the readied mushrooms and the acrid cream five minutes before serving. Heat momentarily and sprinkle with salt and pepper.

This tasty and solid yam nachos recipe contains 47.9 grams of protein and 6.4 grams of fiber in only one serving. These yam nachos are solid, clean, and effectively made paleo and vegetarian, as well. Solid Potato Nachos is a sound option in contrast to customary nachos. This recipe is not difficult to follow and is kid-accommodating as well. All you need is a yam, black beans, chicken, and conventional nacho ingredients to make this fast, simple, fun recipe that is diabetes agreeable, gluten-free, heart-healthy, and low in sodium.

Ingredients:

- 18oz lean meat mince
- 14oz can Mexican-style tomatoes
- 23oz potatoes, daintily cut
- 1 onion, finely cleaved
- 15oz can gentle stew beans
- olive shower oil
- ½ cup ground fat-free cheddar
- To serve
- 2 spring onions, finely slashed
- ⅓ cup fat-free harsh cream
- slashed fresh coriander

Method:

- Preheat broiler to 375°F. Cook potatoes in bubbling water for 8-10 minutes until somewhat delicate.
- 2Brown mince in a non-stick oven. Add onion. Cook for a couple of moments.
- Add beans and tomatoes.
- Cook for 4-5 minutes.
- Mastermind a large portion of the potatoes in a big ovenproof dish or split between 4 person dishes.
- Shower with a little olive oil.
- Spoon over mince. Orchestrate remaining potatoes up and over.
- Splash with oil. Sprinkle with cheddar.
- Prepare for 25 minutes.
- Present with acrid cream, spring onions, and coriander.

48: Sheet Pan Chicken and Brussel Sprouts

This is a real stove-to-table sheet-container supper brimming with delicate, crunchy Brussels sprouts and firm, lemony chicken. A simple lemon-and-spice compound spread sprinkles both the chicken and fledglings, which are then finished off with slender lemon cuts that become crunchy in the broiler, offering a decent textural component and a splendid sprinkle of shading and flavor. The key is to cut the lemon adjusts nearly paper-flimsy, so they can fresh up and lose their harshness.

Ingredients:

- 4 cups Brussels sprouts, quartered

- ¾ teaspoon salt, separated
- ½ teaspoon ground cumin
- ¾ teaspoon ground pepper, separated
- ½ teaspoon dried thyme
- ½ teaspoon dried thyme
- 2 tablespoons extra-virgin olive oil, separated
- 1 pound yams, cut into 1/2-inch wedges
- 1 ¼ pound boneless, skinless chicken thighs, managed

Method:

- Preheat broiler to 425 degrees F.
- Toss yams with 1 tablespoon oil and 1/4 teaspoon each salt and pepper in a large bowl.
- Spread equitably on a rimmed preparing sheet. Broil for 15 minutes.
- Toss Brussels sprouts with the leftover 1 tablespoon oil and 1/4 teaspoon each salt and pepper in the bowl.
- Stir into the yams on the preparing sheet.
- Sprinkle chicken with cumin, thyme, and the leftover 1/4 teaspoon of each salt and pepper. Spot on top of the vegetables.
- Broil until the chicken is cooked through and the vegetables are delicate, 10 to 15 minutes more.
- Move the chicken to a serving platter. Mix vinegar into the vegetables and present with the chicken.

49: Pork Chops with Bloody Mary Tomato Salad

This salad may help you to remember a cocktail or a wedge salad. Consider well drink trims, like celery, parsley, green olives, anchovies, or bacon, when choosing what else to add to this dish.

Ingredients:

- 2 tbsp. red wine vinegar
- 2 tbsp. olive oil
- 2 tsp. Worcestershire sauce
- 1/2 tsp. Tabasco
- 2 tsp. arranged horseradish pressed dry
- 1/2 tsp. celery seeds
- Kosher salt and pepper
- 2 celery stems, daintily cut
- 1-16-ounce cherry tomatoes, split
- 1/2 little red onion, daintily cut
- 1 little head green-leaf lettuce, leaves torn
- 1/4 c. level leaf parsley, finely cleaved
- 4 little bone-in pork slashes (1 in. thick, about 2¼ lbs. all-out)

Method:

- Heat barbecue to medium-high.
- In a big bowl, whisk together oil, vinegar, Worcestershire sauce, horseradish, Tabasco, celery seeds, and ¼ teaspoon salt. Toss with tomatoes, celery, and onion.
- Sprinkle pork slashes with 1/2 teaspoon each salt and pepper and barbecue until brilliant earthy colored and just cooked through, 5 to 7 minutes for every side.
- Overlay parsley into tomatoes and serve over pork and greens.

50: Slow-Cooker Black Eyed Peas

This Slow Cooked Black Eyed Peas recipe requires only a couple of minutes of prep, then everything gets toss in the sluggish cooker! Black peered toward peas are the ideal solace food. Made with an extra ham bone and stewed in a rich delectable stock, these Slow Cooker Black Eyed Peas and Collard Greens are a tasty expansion to your Fresh Year's Day menu.

Ingredients:

- salt, to taste
- 1 shape chicken bouillon
- 6 cups water
- 1 onion, chopped
- 2 cloves garlic, chopped
- 1 pound dried black peered toward peas, arranged and flushed
- 1 jalapeno Chile, cultivated and crushed
- 1 red ringer pepper, stemmed, cultivated, and chopped
- 1 teaspoon ground black pepper
- 8 ounces chopped ham
- 4 cuts bacon, cleaved
- ½ teaspoon cayenne pepper
- 1 ½ teaspoons cumin

Method:

- Empty the water into a lethargic cooker, add the bouillon block, and mix to break down.
- Join the black peered toward peas, onion, salt, Chile pepper, garlic, jalapeno pepper, bacon, cayenne pepper, ham, cumin, and pepper; mix to mix.
- Cover the lethargic cooker and cook on Low for 6 to 8 hours until the beans are delicate.

51: Salmon and Veggies at 5:30 P.M.

Barbecued salmon and veggies make for a beautiful and adjusted fish supper that is prepared in only minutes. The flame broil turns the salmon flaky and sodden while softening the fresh pepper and onion pieces. Balance the supper with earthy-colored rice or quinoa. This carb-cognizant dinner is loaded with protein and nutrients. Transform it into a sheet oven supper recipe if you don't have a meal dish.

Ingredients:

- salt, to taste
- pepper, to taste
- 4 cloves garlic, crushed
- 2 teaspoons ginger
- 4 tablespoons olive oil
- 4 tablespoons lemon juice
- 2 tablespoons fresh thyme
- 2 salmon filets
- 2 lb. little red potato (910 g), or yellow, quartered
- 1 package asparagus, about 1 pound (455g)

Method:

- Preheat the stove to 400°F (200°C).
- Cover a sheet dish with foil or material paper. Spread out potatoes in the oven and sprinkle with olive oil. Sprinkle with salt, pepper, 2 cloves of garlic, and 1 tablespoon lemon juice.
- Heat for 30 minutes.
- Make salmon coating.
- Join salt, pepper, 2 garlic cloves, 1 tablespoon thyme, ginger, 2 tablespoons of olive oil, and 2 tablespoons of lemon juice. Blend well.

- Remove potatoes from the broiler and push them to the top or side of your oven.
- Spot your salmon filets on the container.
- Brush the two sides of the salmon with the coating.
- Spot asparagus on the dish and top with 1 tablespoon olive oil, salt, 1 tablespoon lemon squeeze, and pepper.
- Sprinkle 1 tsp of thyme on the potatoes and asparagus.
- Prepare for 10-12 minutes. (The salmon should piece effectively with a fork when it's prepared.) Enjoy!

52: Poached Egg with Asparagus and Tomato

This supper is a fast and simple path for any recipe phobe to prepare an overly scrumptious dish in a matter of moments. With their various medical advantages, eggs are extraordinary at any time and taste scrumptious when presented with fresh asparagus lances.

Ingredients:

- 1 tablespoon honey
- 1 tablespoon Dijon mustard
- 2 shallots, shaved slight
- ½ cup olive oil
- 1 lemon, supreme, and juiced*
- Coarse salt and fresh broke pepper, to taste
- 2 garlic cloves, crushed
- 2 packages asparagus, bottoms managed
- 4 Creole tomatoes, cut in thick adjusts
- 6 tablespoons parmesan, ground
- 4 eggs

Method:

- Carry a big pot of salted water to stew and keep prepared.
- In the mixing bowl, add Dijon mustard, shallots, honey, lemon Supremes, and juice. Race in olive oil and sprinkle with salt and pepper. Put dressing in a safe spot.
- In the large oven, add a sprinkle of olive oil and singe asparagus stems in clumps with a spot of crushed garlic. Sprinkle with salt and pepper.
- Spot stems in a single layer in the oven so they don't steam and overcook.
- If planning early, place promptly into the cooler, serve chilled.
- Have everything plated and all set before poaching eggs, as they are time-touchy.
- On large plates mastermind cuts of tomato, marginally covering one another.
- Shower tomatoes with olive oil and sprinkle with salt and pepper.
- Gap and organize singed asparagus on plates.
- To poach eggs, add a sprinkle of white vinegar to a pot of stewing water.
- Whirl spoon around in your water to make it move in roundabout movement and afterward break and drop your eggs into the center.
- Delicately twirl water.
- Poach 2-4 minutes to cook, or until whites are firm to contact and focus are giggly.
- To gather, place one poached egg on top of each heap of asparagus.
- Blend vinaigrette and delicately spoon over the egg, asparagus, and tomatoes.

- Get done with freshly ground parmesan and serve right away.

53: Yogurt with Blueberries

A simple blend of Greek yogurt and blueberries gets an additional dash of pleasantness from brilliant honey. It's the ideal equilibrium of protein and fiber to keep you empowered. These two food varieties draw out the best in one another.

The high fiber substance of the berries (just about four grams for every cup) reinforces the sound microbes found in yogurt, also known as probiotics, assisting it with enduring the dangerous excursion through the stomach-related lot. Once in the gut, the probiotics assist the body with engrossing the solvent fiber of the blueberries.

Ingredients:

- ¼ cup blueberries
- 1 cup nonfat plain Greek yogurt

Method:

- Spot yogurt in a bowl and top with blueberries.

54: Feta and Tomato Omelets

Add the Mediterranean contort to your plate with this Feta and Tomato Omelets recipe with feta cheddar, black olives, and tomato. Greek omelet is an exceptionally flexible dish one can appreciate at any time. It very well may be filled in as a filling high-energy breakfast, a quick bite with some dry town bread, or even dinner.

This Feta and Tomato Omelets recipe is truly simple to plan and incorporates basic ingredients, however, the taste is truly flawless and fresh. You will adore the blend of feta and tomato.

Ingredients:

- 3 black Kalamata olives
- 1/2 tomato, slashed into shapes
- 60g/2 oz. feta cheddar disintegrated
- 2 tbsps. olive oil
- a squeeze dried oregano
- 3 large eggs
- ground Graviera cheddar to decorate
- salt and freshly ground pepper

Method:

- To make this heavenly Greek omelet recipe start by setting up the ingredients first.
- Remove the seeds and add juice from the tomato and cut the tissue into little 3D squares. Put in a safe spot.
- Remove the pits from the olives and cut them into little pieces. Put in a safe spot.

- Disintegrate the feta cheddar with your hands or utilizing a fork and set it aside.
- Break the eggs in a bowl and sprinkle with salt and pepper. Beat the eggs with a fork until consolidated.
- Heat a little medium nonstick griddle over medium heat.
- Add 2 tbsps. olive oil and the beaten eggs. Utilizing a spatula, drag the omelet towards the one finish of the oven and slant the dish to allow the crude eggs to fill the unfilled side.
- Rehash this interaction for approx. 1-2 minutes until the omelet is cooked. (the eggs are set yet the top is still marginally clammy)
- Remove the dish from the heat and add the tomato, feta cheddar, olives, oregano.
- Slip the spatula under the omelet, tip to release, and delicately overlay the omelet fifty-fifty.
- Sprinkle with ground cheddar and serve.

55: Spicy Chocolate Keto Fat Bombs

Keto chocolate is high in fat and sugar-free for a low carb contort, however all you'll taste is smooth, velvety dull chocolate flavor combined with an impactful zest blend that makes certain to warm you up a bit! It's so natural to make chocolate at home with only a couple of ingredients.

Try it and see with your own eyes. These scrumptious and delish keto fat bombs make certain to be hit. Fill in as keto pastries, keto snacks, keto sweet treat, or make to take to parties. These are even raved about by people who don't follow a ketogenic diet/lifestyle.

You can add a wide range of additional ingredients to the focal point of the hot cocoa bombs, sprinkles to the outside, or considerably more dissolved chocolate. They look so extravagant and beautiful, so normally, they are stunning endowments as well.

Ingredients:

- ⅓ cup cocoa powder
- ½ cup sugar
- ⅓ cup weighty cream powder
- 7 oz. ChocZero sugar free chocolate chips (1 sack of milk or dim chips)

Optional:

- sugar free sprinkles
- 1 tsp coconut oil
- ¼ cup ChocZero without sugar white chocolate chips

Method:

- Microwave the sugar free chocolate chips for 30 seconds.
- Mix. If they aren't softened microwave at 15 seconds spans, mixing after each.
- When they are about 75% softened simply mix until they are liquefied.
- Spoon a stacking teaspoon into every cavity of a 2-inch circle form. Utilize the rear of the teaspoon to push the chocolate up the edges.
- As it sets keep pushing chocolate up the sides to make a thicker shell.
- Spot a storing tablespoon of the hot cocoa blend inside a large portion of the circles.
- Spoon on dissolved chocolate around the edge.
- Top with the second 50% of the circle.

- Optional: Drizzle with extra liquefied chocolate blended in with 1 teaspoon of coconut oil and top with sprinkles.
- Refrigerate until fixed.
- Spot a hot cocoa bomb into a mug.
- Pour 6-ounce of hot milk on chocolate bomb.
- Mix until smooth.

Conclusion:

Thus, in conclusion, just by following a two times per week 24-hour Intermittent fasting plan for half a month you will get a healthy and slim body. However, if you can improve your diet when that you don't fast then you will lose more weight, and assuming you can adhere to this system, you will keep the load off without falling back on any accident diets or diets that are only difficult to adhere to.

Intermittent fasting has been appeared to reduce the kind of white platelet called monocytes. Monocytes are connected with body irritation. By reducing inflammation, constant musculoskeletal agonies can be improved. Cancer cells ordinarily feed on glucose. Blood glucose is high when we nibble and eat much of the time. Alternately, when we fast Intermittently, we burn fat.

Since most cancer cells can't benefit from fat disease hazard exercises. A few studies show that Intermittent fasting helps the body with clearing out toxins and harmed cells. This purifying and refinement lessens sleepiness and languor and helps support energy.

When starting with Intermittent fasting, make sure you start simple, getting your body used to avoiding a day once per week, then maybe two. Also, go slowly when working out during this changing time, until you begin to feel like you're ready to take a full burden in your exercise program. This will not take long, and indeed, will leave you wanting more.

If you're looking for a way to speed up your fat loss and continue to work out, then you need to investigate Intermittent fasting. You might be satisfied with exactly how compelling it tends to be at easily lessening your caloric intake while letting your adequate energy finish your exercises.

For somebody who is sound and needs to attempt Intermittent fasting, it should not be troublesome. Nonetheless, people with dietary problems, diabetes, diseases, people who are finished or underweight should counsel certified health proficient before beginning with this kind of eating pattern.

To conclude, we need to comprehend that Intermittent fasting is not a magic pill. A certified nutritionist can fabricate a successful weight management program with Intermittent fasting by consolidating a sound diet of nutritious genuine food sources with customary exercise and satisfactory rest.

KETO DIET

The Comprehensive Guide For Weight Loss, to Heal Your body and feel good.

Introduction

As modern problems need a modern solution, and the same approach is required to deal with modern health diseases like cancer, obesity, heart disease, and alike. The introduction of new technology has provided immense ease to humanity, reducing workforce application for carrying out laborious tasks. The introduction of new powerful, multi-purpose, and easy to use machines has replaced humans working in various workspace fields. There are certain classes of people for whom technology has proven to be more beneficial than they have imagined. Simultaneously, there is a wide extended class of people who have lost their job and are suffering from earning their livelihood.

Furthermore, there exists a class whose workload has been decreased while they are retaining their job. Workspace for the latter described class has mostly been restricted to a single chair from where they deal with their respective computers to perform their assigned tasks throughout their extensive working hours. Although their workload has been decreased compared to the past, they had to perform tasks using physical energy, which indirectly helped them remain physically fit while maintaining good health. Their job was a sort of exercise. However, they are at more because they are at ease physically, and their physical workload is taken upon by machines. This ease has not reduced their work hours, and they had to work for an extended time that does not allows them to make out some time for themselves to exercise regularly to maintain their physical and mental health. Nowadays, people are more prone to diseases, and due to changes in surroundings, new diseases are finding ground making people remain more conscious about their health. Obesity is one of the most commonly reported diseases nowadays. Patients complain of an increase in their weight, swelling of their belly, and misalignment of their body structure, making them look ugly and unconfident. Once this disease reaches its climax, it triggers several other diseases like heart disease, blood pressure variation, diabetes and many more. Technology has always helped human beings counter their problem, so in this case, there are certain methods to easily get rid of this disease. The Keto diet is one of the most appreciated techniques to increase weight problems with no side effects. Keto diet focuses on curbing the intake of carbohydrate and allowing a moderate level of protein while encouraging fat intake because food intake with this kind of nutrition will change the metabolic pathway of extracting energy from glucose breakdown to breakdown of stored fats which in turn will cause a reduction in weight of an individual. This diet includes a meal plan in which different dishes are proposed for a patient whose ingredients are measured according to the nutrients mentioned above. This will help the patient to burn their fat quickly without providing room for their replacement, hence triggering the weight loss without much hard work. This technique demands determination and discipline to follow the diet plan religiously; otherwise, patients may have to suffer its side effects.

KETO DIET
FOOD PYRAMID

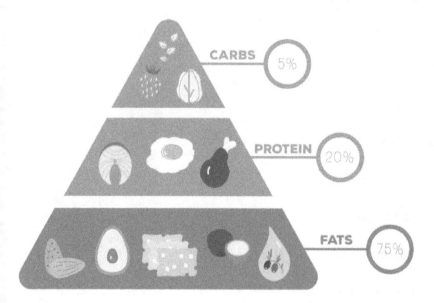

CARBS 5%

PROTEIN 20%

FATS 75%

Chapter 1: Breakfast Recipes

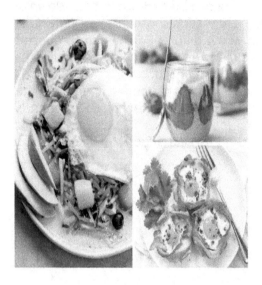

1. Breakfast Casserole

Ready in: 85 mins

Servings: 12

Difficulty: Difficult

INGREDIENTS

- 2 cup shredded ham

- Salt to taste

- Pepper to taste

- 1 tsp season salt

- 1 ½ cup grated jack cheese

- 12 eggs

- 24 oz chopped potatoes

- 1 ½ cup grated cheddar cheese

DIRECTIONS

1. Add pepper and salt in chopped and frozen potatoes and pour in a pan.

2. Take another bowl, whisk eggs in it and then add all the remaining ingredients.

3. Pour it over the frozen potatoes and refrigerate overnight.

4. Heat the oven at 350°C and bake it for 90 minutes.

5. Serve and enjoy it.

NUTRITION: Calories: 225 kcal Fat: 18 g Protein: 14 g Carbohydrates: 2 g

2. Onion Omelet

Ready in: 10 minutes

Servings: 2

Difficulty: Easy

INGREDIENTS

- White pepper to taste

- Three eggs

- 1 tsp soy sauce

- 1tpsp oyster sauce

- Sesame oil (sprinkle)

- 2tpsp cooking oil

- One diced onions

DIRECTIONS

1. Take a bowl to add pepper, salt, sesame oil, oyster, and soya sauce.

2. Add finely chopped onion and mix it.

3. Cook each side for 3 minutes.

4. Serve and enjoy.

NUTRITION: Calories: 240 cal Fat: 18.4 g Protein: 14 g Carbs: 4.6 g

3. Bacon and Eggs

Ready in: 20 minutes

Servings: 4

Difficulty: Easy

INGREDIENTS

- 150 g bacon

- Salt taste

- Pepper to taste

- Eight eggs

- ¼ cup parsley

- ½ cup tomatoes

DIRECTIONS

1. Take a pan and fry bacon over medium to low heat.

2. Cook eggs in a separate pan with a sunny side up, and then add tomatoes to it.

3. Add the seasoning you want and serve it hot.

NUTRITION: Calories: 370 kcal Fat: 31 g Protein: 20 g Carbs: 1 g

4. Eggs with Ham

Ready in: 20 minutes

Servings: 4

Difficulty: Easy

INGREDIENTS

- 1 cup cheese, shredded

- ¼ cup olive oil

- One minced jalapeno pepper

- Eight beaten eggs

- Pepper to taste

- Salt to taste

- 3tbsp milk

- ½ cup finely chopped ham

- ¼ cup salt

DIRECTIONS

1. Take a bowl and beat eggs, black pepper, seasoned salt, and salt in it.

2. Sauté jalapeno in olive oil over medium flame for 3 to 4 mins.

3. Then add ham to it and cook for 2 mins.

4. Pour the mixture of egg in jalapeno mixture and cook for 4 to 5 mins.

5. Sprinkle half cheese over it and cook till cheese melts.

6. Turn off the flame and add the remaining amount of cheese over it.

7. Serve and enjoy.

NUTRITION: Calories: 400 cal Fat: 33 g Protein: 23 g Carbs: 1.8 g

5. Chia Oatmeal

Prep time: 5 minutes

Chill time: 8 hours

Servings: 1

Difficulty: Difficult

INGREDIENTS

- One sliced banana

- ¼ tsp vanilla

- ¾ cup almond milk, unsweetened

- 2tbsp almonds, sliced and toasted

- 1/3 cup oats

- 2 tsp honey

- 2tbsp cranberries, dried

- 1tbsp chia seeds

DIRECTIONS

1. Combine all the ingredients in a mixing bowl.

2. Stir the mixture thoroughly and refrigerate it overnight.

3. Garnish with almonds and banana before serving.

NUTRITION: Calories: 485 cal Fat: 15 g Protein: 10 g Carbs: 85 g

6. Curry Cauliflower Rice Bowls

Ready in: 15 mins

Servings: 4

Difficulty: Easy

INGREDIENTS

- ½ cup green peas

- 3tbsp olive oil

- 12 oz. cauliflower rice

- ½ cup chopped bell pepper (red)

- ¼ tablespoon ground coriander

- ½ cup chopped onion

- Salt to taste

- ½ cup chopped onion, Sweet

- 1 ½ tablespoon curry powder

- Two crushed garlic cloves

- ¼tbsp turmeric powder

DIRECTIONS

1. Sauté onion and bell pepper in a pan for 5-6 mins in olive oil.

2. Then add garlic powder in it and sauté it for 2 mins.

3. Take a bowl and mix salt, curry powder, coriander, and turmeric.

4. Add peas, seasoning mix, and cauliflower rice in the pan and cook it for 7-8 mins over medium flame.

5. Serve and enjoy.

NUTRITION: Calories: 101 kcal Fat: 7.5 g Protein: 2.9 g Carbs: 5 g

7. Pesto Scrambled Eggs

Ready in: 10 minutes

Servings: 1

Difficulty: Easy

INGREDIENTS

- ½ tsp pesto

- 1tbsp oil

- Salt as required

- Pepper as required

- One beaten egg

- ½ cup cheese, shredded

DIRECTIONS

1. Combine all the ingredients in a bowl.

2. Pour this mixture into the pan and cook it for 5-6 mins over medium flame with continuous stirring.

3. Turn off the flame and stir it in pesto.

NUTRITION: Calories: 319 cal Fat: 29.1 g Protein: 13.8 g Carbs: 0.9 g

8. Egg and Mushroom Breakfast

Ready in: 10 mins

Servings: 3

Difficulty: Easy

INGREDIENTS

- ½ cup onion, chopped

- Two eggs

- Pepper as required

- Salt as required

- 2tbsp olive oil

- Parsley

DIRECTIONS

1. Sauté onions in a pan over medium flame.

2. Then add mushrooms in it and cook for 5-6 mins.

3. Take a bowl, beat eggs in it and then add black pepper and salt it.

4. Pour this mixture into the pan and cook for 5-8 mins.

5. When eggs are cooked, remove heat and serve it.

NUTRITION: Calories: 186.9 cal Fat: 14.3 g Protein: 12 g Carbs: 12 g

9. Cheesy Sausage Potatoes

Ready in: 20 minutes

Servings: 8

Difficulty: Easy

INGREDIENTS

- 2 cups cheese

- One chopped onion

- 3 lb. potatoes, sliced

- ¼ cup butter

- 1 lb. pork sausage

DIRECTIONS

1. Boil potatoes in a pan, then reduce the flame and simmer them for 7-8 mins.

2. Take another pan, add onion and crumbled sausage. Cook till meat is fully cooked.

3. Now add sausage mixture and potatoes in a baking dish and top with cheese.

4. Bake this mixture at 350° for 8 mins.

NUTRITION: Calories: 252 cal Fat: 13 g Protein: 9 g Carbs: 26 g

10. Almond and Strawberry Oatmeal

Ready in: 8 minutes

Servings: 1

Difficulty: Easy

INGREDIENTS

- Strawberries

- 1 cup water or milk

- ¼ tsp vanilla extract

- ½ cup oats

- Salt to taste

- Few almonds

- ½ banana

- ½ tsp almond extract

DIRECTIONS

1. Boil milk in a pan and add oats to it over medium flame.

2. Add mashed banana to the pan.

3. After few minutes, add salt, vanilla, and almond extract and stir it.

4. Now add sliced strawberries into oatmeal.

5. Keep on heating till the desired consistency is obtained.

6. Add desired toppings and serve them.

NUTRITION: Calories: 282 cal Fat: 12.4 g Protein: 5.6 g Carbs: 33.9 g

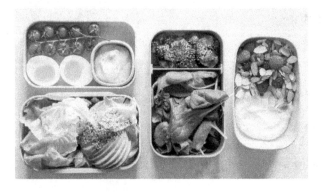

1. Curry Pork and Kale

Ready in: 25 minutes

Servings: 5

Difficulty: Easy

INGREDIENTS

- One onion

- One packet of brown lentils

- 240 g pork

- One packet tomato

- One container pasanda seasoning

- 200 ml coconut milk

- One packet ginger

- One green onion

- One packet chicken broth crumb

- 2 Naan

- 100 g kale

DIRECTIONS

1. Preheat your 400 Fahrenheit oven. Heat a drizzle of oil over med to high heat in a frying pan.

2. Add the ground pork when hot and season with salt and pepper. Cook for 4-5 mins, until golden brown. To break it up as it cooks, use a wooden spoon.

3. Halve the peel and slice the onion thinly when the pork is browning.

4. The garlic is peeled and rubbed

5. Drain and rinse these lentils in a sieve.

6. Stir in the onion until the pork is browned. Cook until softened, 4-5 mins with the pork mince. Stir in the garlic, pasanda pepper, tomato puree, and ginger puree. Mix and cook for 1 min, then add coconut milk, water, and powdered chicken stock. Stir in the lentils, bring to a boil and simmer until slightly reduced 3-4 mins.

7. Meanwhile, cut and thinly slice the spring onion.

8. Into the pork mixture, mix the kale.

9. Cover with a cap or some tin foil and cook for 3-4 mins until the kale is tender. Meanwhile, to heat up, pop the naan into your oven for 3-4 mins.

10. Taste the curry and season with salt and pepper.

NUTRITION: Calories: 874 kcal Fat: 39.0 g Protein: 42 g Carbs: 85 g

2. Mustard and Rosemary Pork Chops with Swiss Chard

Ready in: 30 minutes

Servings: 4

Difficulty: Easy

INGREDIENTS

- 2 tbsp mustard

- Four pork lions, cubes

- 1 tbsp butter

- 3 tbsp breadcrumbs

- 1 tbsp rosemary

- Two dried garlic

- 1/2 cup onion, chopped.

- 1 tbsp honey

- 1 Swiss cluster chard

- 1 tsp lemon

- 2 tsp wine vinegar

DIRECTIONS

1.   Preheat the oven and place a rack in the top third of the oven to broil. Powder the pork with half of the salt and pepper on both sides. In a large oven-safe skillet, heat half of the butter over a med pan and cook the pork until golden, 3 to 4 mins. Remove from the heat, brush tops with mustard, then scatter uniformly overtop with rosemary and breadcrumbs. Place the skillet beneath the broiler till the pork is fried and golden, around 2 mins.

2.   Meanwhile, over moderate melt, heat the remaining butter in a broad deep-sided frying pan. Add the onion, garlic, and chard stem and simmer for 2 to 3 mins, until tender.

3.   Stir in the chard leaves and 30 mL of water. Season with salt and pepper to taste, cover and simmer until tender, about 5 mins.

NUTRITION: Calories: 230 kcal Fat: 7 g Protein: 27 g Carbs: 14 g

3. Pork Fried Cauliflower Rice

Ready in: 25 minutes

Servings: 5

Difficulty: Easy

INGREDIENTS

- Salt to taste

- 2 tsp sesame oil

- 1 lb pork

- 2 cups cabbage

- Pepper to taste

- Four sliced onion

- One sliced carrot

- 2 tsp sliced ginger

- Four bulbs of garlic, sliced

- 2 tbsp soy sauce

- 4 cups cauliflower rice

DIRECTIONS

1. In a med saucepan, heat the sesame seed. Add pork and cook until heated through and no longer green, breaking it up as it heats. It's going to take 6-8 mins.

2. Cabbage, onions, green onion, garlic, and ginger are added. Once the cabbage and carrots are tender, simmer for 4-5 mins.

3. Stir in the rice from the cauliflower and press it into the pan. Let it cook without changing it for 3-4 mins before the rice starts to brown. Mix and repeat then.

4. Stir in the sauce with the soy. As required, taste and add more soy sauce.

NUTRITION: Calories: 286 kcal Fat: 12 g Protein: 27 g Carbs: 13 g

4. Asian Pork Meatballs with Noodles and Vegetable Rice

Ready in: 30 minutes

Servings: 2

Difficulty: Easy

INGREDIENTS

- One slice ginger

- Three onion

One lime

One bulbs garlic

1 cluster coriander

One carrot

- ½ package Rice Noodle

One bunch coriander

- 3 tbsp soy sauce

- 250 g pork mince

- One packet Mangetout

- 15 g Breadcrumbs

25 g peanuts

- 2 tbsp soy sauce

DIRECTIONS

1. Thinly slice the root and cut it from the spring onion. Peel the ginger and garlic and finely grind them. Zest and cut the lime in two. Remove the carrot ends and grate coarsely. Chop the coriander loosely. Make the kettle boil.

2. Placed them in a bowl with the rice noodles. To fully submerge them, spill sufficiently hot water over the noodles, then cover them with cling film or a pan. Leave to the side before depleting in a colander for 8-10 mins

3. In a mixing cup, pop the pork mince and add half of the garlic, half of the spring onion, half of the ginger, and all of the lime zest. Add a fourth of the amount of soy to all the panko breadcrumbs and mix well to combine. Shape the mixture into four meatballs for every person.

4. Heat a drizzle of oil over med to high heat in a large cooking pot. Add the meatballs and fry, rotating periodically, 8-10 mins, until browned all over. Add the remaining spring onion, ginger, and garlic along with the mange tout and carrot until the meatballs are golden brown, then stir-fry all for 1 min.

5. Add the ketchup and leftover soy sauce, mix and boil for 2-3 mins, then tip in the noodles and half the coriander. Squeeze half of the lime into the juice. Toss until the noodles are piping hot to mix and heat,2-3 mins.

6. Serve it in sprinkle and bowls over the rest of the coriander and the peanuts. With a slice of the remaining lime, serve.

NUTRITION: Calories: 686 kcal Fat: 27.0 g Protein: 36 g Carbs: 76 g

5. Jalapeno-Garlic-Onion Cheeseburgers

Ready in: 25 minutes

Servings: 4

Difficulty: Easy

INGREDIENTS

- ½ cup sliced jalapeno
- 2 tbsp garlic
- One chopped onion
- 1 lb beef
- 1 cup jack cheese
- Four hamburger buns

DIRECTIONS

1. Heat the grill pan over high heat.
2. Take a bowl and mix pepper, onion, ground beef, and garlic in it. Make small patties from it.
3. Grill the patties for 3-5 minutes and top with cheese.
4. Serve with buns.
5. Enjoy.

NUTRITION: Calories: 474 Cal Fat: 26.8 g Protein: 31.6 g Carbs: 24.8 g

6. Jalapeno Popper Chicken

Ready in: 35 minutes

Servings: 6

Difficulty: Easy

INGREDIENTS

- 1.5 lb chicken boneless
- salt & pepper
- 8 oz cream cheese
- 2 tbsps milk
- 1/2 tsp garlic powder
- ½ cup chopped jalapeno peppers
- 1/2 cup of cooked bacon
- 1 cup of cheddar

DIRECTIONS

1.   Take the baking dish & spray it with oil.

2.   Put the chicken in layers over the baking dish and season with salt & pepper.

3.   Take a bowl and mix garlic powder, cheese, and cream at room temperature.

4.   Spread the mixture on chicken and sprinkle cheese, peppers, and bacon over it.

5. Cover the dish with aluminum foil and bake for 35-40 minutes.

6. Serve and enjoy.

NUTRITION: Calories: 349 Cal Fat: 26 g Protein: 28 g Carbs: 1 g

7. Perfect Sirloin Beef Roast

Ready in: 1 hour 45 minutes

Servings: 12

Difficulty: Difficult

INGREDIENTS

- 7 lb beef sirloin roast

- One onion

- Two celery ribs

- Two carrots

- 3 tbsp garlic

- 1/2 cup of water

Spice mix

- 3 tbsp onion flakes

- 2 tbsp oregano

- 1 tbsp peppercorns

- 1 tbsp coriander

- 1 tbsp Himalayan salt

- 1½ tsp chili pepper flakes

DIRECTIONS

1. Grind the spices & mix.

2. Clean the meat and spread spices over it. Cover the meat with plastic and put it in the fridge for one whole day.

3. Take a baking dish and put onion, carrot, garlic and celery, and some water in it. Place the meat over it.

4. Bake it in preheated oven for 10-15 minutes.

6. Put aluminum foil and roast in the oven for more than 30 minutes.

7. Take out the dish from the oven and place it over the cutting board.

8. Remove the carve.

9. Serve and enjoy.

NUTRITION: Calories: 312 Cal Fat: 8 g Protein: 53 g Carbs: 3 g

3. Country Fried Steak

Ready in: 20 minutes

Servings: 6

Difficulty: Easy

INGREDIENTS

One 1/2lbs steak

- 1 cup of all-purpose flour

- 1 tsp paprika

- 1 1/2 tsp salt

1 1/4 tsp pepper

Butter

2 1/2 cups milk

Three eggs

4 tbsp oil

DIRECTIONS

1. Take 3-4 bowls and put eggs and half a cup of milk with one flour cup.

2. Mix one tbsp of salt and pepper along with paprika in the flour mixture.

3. Dip the steaks in milk first and then in the flour mixture.

4. Now dip the steaks in eggs and again into the flour.

5. Take a large skillet and heat a small amount of olive oil over medium flame.

6. Fry the steaks in the skillet for 10-15 minutes till they get brown color.

7. Melt the butter with a small amount of oil in the pan.

8. Add milk and stir continuously till it gets a boil and becomes thick.

9. Remove it from the stove.

10. Serve the steaks with gravy and mashed potatoes.

11. Enjoy.

NUTRITION: Calories: 272.2 Cal Fat: 139 g Protein: 9.1 g Carbs: 24.2 g

9. Asian Pork Meatballs

Ready in: 60 minutes

Servings: 5

Difficulty: Medium

INGREDIENTS

- 3 tbsp fish sauce

- 2 tbsp honey

- One bulb chopped garlic

- Four crushed onion

- 1 tsp cornflour

- 2 tsp crushed lemongrass

- 2 tbsp crushed coriander

- 1 tbsp crushed mint

- For sauce

- 1 tsp crushed coriander

- 2 tbsp lemon juice

- Three chopped onion

- 1 tsp sesame oil

- 2 tbsp soy sauce

DIRECTIONS

1. Make meatballs. In a non-stick frying pan, melt the honey softly, add the fish sauce and stir to make a syrup.

2. In a bowl, put the pork and add in the honey syrup, green onions, garlic, lemongrass, cornflower, mint, and cilantro. Add salt and black pepper to the blend and season.

3. Make it 20 balls and place them on a paper-lined tray, 30 mins to relax. All the ingredients are combined to make the sauce and put aside.

4. Brush the olive oil on the balls and fry each side for 3-4 mins. Serve.

NUTRITION: Calories: 51 kcal Fat: 3 g Protein: 5 g Carbs: 3 g

10. Eggplant and Chili Garlic Port Stir Fry

Ready in: 30 minutes

Servings: 4

Difficulty: Easy

INGREDIENTS

- 1 lb eggplant

- 3 tbsp olive oil

- Three bulbs garlic

- ½ chopped onion,

- One zucchini

- ½ lb pork

- 2 tbsp fish sauce

- 2 tbsp garlic sauce

- Black pepper to taste

- 1 tbsp rice vinegar

DIRECTIONS

1. Over med-high heat, heat a skillet. Add two tsp of olive oil, then add the eggplant to the mixture. Cook for 3-5 min until the eggplant is seared, rotating periodically. Take the eggplant outside the pan and move it aside.

2. Then add the remaining olive oil to the skillet, and stir in the garlic and onions. Heat until soft, and then stir in the ground pork for 1 min or until soft. Cook until the pork is browned, or around 3 min.

3. Mix in the zucchini, sauce with chili garlic, sauce with fish, and vinegar with rice. Cook till the zucchini is soft, about 3 mins. Mix in the eggplant and continue to cook for 2 mins or until some of the eggplant sauce has been drained by heating and frying.

NUTRITION: Calories: 452 kcal Fat: 23 g Protein: 29.8 g Carbs: 33.3 g

11. Thai Shrimp and Eggplant Stir Fry

Ready in: 34 minutes

Servings: 4

Difficulty: Medium

INGREDIENTS

- 1 ½ tbsp fish sauce

- 2 tbsp lemon juice

- 5 tsp peanut oil

- 1 ½ tsp sugar

- Three eggplants

- 1 lb shrimp

- Two chilies

- Five bulbs garlic

- 1 cup basil leaves

- One sliced spring onion

- Rice noodles, cooked.

- Slice of lime wedges

DIRECTIONS

1. Whisk the fish sauce, sugar, lime juice, and water in a small dish.

2. Heat 1 tbsp oil on med heat until quite hot in a 12-inches non-stick skillet; swirl to cover the skillet. Add shrimp and stir-fry for about 3 mins.

3. Into the skillet and half of the eggplant, add oil. Cook for an additional min, uninterrupted, then stir-fry for 30 secs. Move it to a shrimp dish. Add two additional tsp. Of oil; repeat for remaining eggplant. In the middle, make a well and add the remaining oil, garlic, chili, and scallion—Stir-fry for around 1 min.

4. To the skillet, add the lobster, eggplant, and sauce. Cook, toss well until fully heated 30 sec-1 min. Serve with rice noodles and lime wedges.

NUTRITION: Calories: 209 kcal Fat: 10 g Protein: 18 g Carbs: 12 g

12. Lemon Chicken with Artichokes and Kale

Ready in: 25 minutes

Servings: 1

Difficulty: Easy

INGREDIENTS

- 3 tbsp olive oil

- 6 oz kale

- ½ tsp black pepper

- 5 oz chicken

- 9 oz artichokes

- ¼ tsp salt

- 1 tbsp decide thyme,

- One lemon

- ¼ tsp red pepper powder

- 2 oz cheese

DIRECTIONS

1. With the oven rack in the top spot, preheat the broiler to high. In the oven, put a rimmed baking dish.

2. In a cup, combine the kale and 1 tbsp oil; rub the leaves until slightly wilted with your fingertips.

3. Sprinkle black salt and pepper with the chicken. Take the pan from the oven very carefully. To the plate, add 1 tbsp of oil; turn the pan to coat. Add the chicken to the saucepan; boil for five mins.

4. Add the artichokes and pieces of lemon to the pan. Sprinkle oil and thyme. Broil before you're done with chicken, 10 to 12 mins. Place the chicken on a cutting panel. Add the kale mixture to the pan; broil for 3 to 5 mins until the kale is fried and the sides are crisp.

5. Send the chicken back to the pan; add cheese, lemon juice, thyme, and pepper.

NUTRITION: Calories: 417 kcal Fat: 19 g Protein: 40 g Carbs: 20 g

13. Crispy Roast Duck with Fennel and Orange

Ready in: 75 minutes

Servings: 5

Difficulty: difficult

INGREDIENTS

- One orange

- 1 Duck

- One bottle cider

- One fennel, slice into 8th pieces

- ¼ cup chopped apricots

- 1 cup chicken soup

- 2 tbsp sugar

- Four spring thyme

- Olive oil

- Salt to taste

DIRECTIONS

1. To 400 Fahrenheit, pre-heat the oven.

2. Set the duck down on the other side of the skin of an oven tray. Place the orange with some sea salt inside the duck cavity. Place the mixture in the oven and prepare it for 30 mins. Switch to the side of the skin after 30 mins and cook for another hour.

3. Place all the remaining ingredients in the pan and bake for 45 minutes.

4. If the fennel has been braised, cut it, keep it warm and pass the liquid to a saucepan. Add the starch, bring it to a boil, and simmer. Reduce to a clotted sauce and to serve, set aside.

5. Carve the breast and the legs out of the duck to serve. Cut the breasts and place them next to the braised fennel on a platter.

NUTRITION: Calories: 514 kcal Fat: 43 g Protein: 15 g Carbs: 18 g

14. Duck Chili

Ready in: 80 minutes

Servings: 6

Difficulty: difficult

INGREDIENTS

- 3 tbsp duck Fat
- 1 Duck Breast
- 1/8 cup chopped chili
- One crushed onion
- 1 tbsp chopped garlic
- 1 tbsp cumin
- Three chopped carrots
- ½ tbsp oregano
- 1 tbsp paprika
- 1 cup beef broth
- 8 oz tomato juice
- 9 oz kidney beans
- 1 tbsp vinegar

- 1 cup crushed mushrooms

- One crushed green pepper

DIRECTIONS

1. Grind the duck breast by hand. Put for 5 mins in the fridge. Remove the substance and grind it with a small knife. Break the duck breast into thin slices across the width and then again across the thickness. Chopping until you have a clean, coarse grind is the final stage.

2. In a deep dutch oven, melt the duck fat over med-low heat and add the onion—Cook for 10 mins, or till your potatoes are tender. Alternatively, you might make this duck chili dish in a crockpot or slow cooker.

3. Cook for 5 mins after adding the garlic and carrots.

4. Flakes of red pepper, cumin, paprika, chili powder, and oregano are added. Then, prepare 3 mins of duck chili. Next, add broth, tomato sauce, and vinegar. Stir, then cook for 40 mins and cover.

5. Mushrooms and bell peppers are added. Let the duck chili boil for 15 more mins. Immediately serve.

NUTRITION: Calories: 340 kcal Fat: 8 g Protein: 19 g Carbs: 51 g

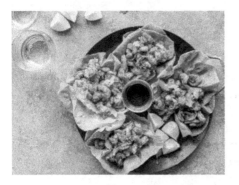

1. Beer and Mushroom Instant Pot Roast

Ready in: 140 minutes

Servings: 6

Difficulty: Difficult

INGREDIENTS

- 3 cups onion soup

- 4 lb Blade Roast

- One sliced onion

- 2 tbsp olive oil

- 2 Stalks celery

- 1 tsp sauce

- 1 tbsp garlic paste

- 10.75 oz mushroom soup

2 cup bottle wine

10 oz mushroom

DIRECTIONS

.   Here for this recipe, the instant pot is used. Olive oil is added to it and turns it on. After burning roast in it, turn off the instant pot.

.   Then all available vegetables are added.

.   Different ingredients like beer, Worcestershire sauce, and soup are mixed in a measuring cup.

.   Then this mixture is poured on the roast.

.   For almost two hours, cook the roast by turning on the instant pot's meat button while keeping in view that pressure should be high.

.   Release steam produced in the pot it could be done manually or naturally as well.

.   Then take a saucepan and add pour sauce in it (about 2-3 cups). Boil it for u5 to 6 minutes.

.   And then, take one teaspoon of cornstarch to add it to a quarter cup of water. Pour it on the boiling sauce and cook it for a time.

.   Roast beef is ready and serves to guests along with tasty gravy.

NUTRITION: Calories: 324 kcal Fat: 21 g Protein: 29 g Carbs: 2 g

2. Coconut Pork Curry

Ready in: 4 hours 40 minutes

Servings: 8

Difficulty: Difficult

INGREDIENTS

- 3 cups chicken soup

- 2 tbsp oil

- One sliced of onion

- 4 lb boneless pork

- Salt to taste

- 1 tbsp Grained curry powder

- Black pepper to taste

- 1 cup coconut milk

- Three cloves chopped Garlic

- 14 oz chopped tomatoes

- 3 tbsp chopped ginger

- ½ tsp turmeric powder

- Boil rice

DIRECTIONS

1. First of all, olive oil is heated in a skillet. Pork is flavored by mixing with table salt pepper. Divide the pork into two halves, add one of them in the skillet and cook it for about 12-15 minutes at moderate heat. Then similarly transfer the other half and brown it.

2. Then add 2 tbsp of fat to this browned pork skillet. Add certain other ingredients like garlic, curry, onion, cumin, and turmeric, and cook it at low heat. Continue stirring while cooking until you feel their fragrance. Separate all this mixture into a slow cooker. To make it tastier, add coconut milk, tomatoes, and tomato juice and then cook it in a small cooker for about 4 hours. Remove fat from the surface of stew. Your recipe is ready to serve it elegantly to your guests.

NUTRITION: Calories: 491 kcal Fat: 25 g Protein: 46 g Carbs: 21 g

3. Buffalo Pulled Pork with Bacon

Ready in: 4 Hours 10 minutes

Servings: 10

Difficulty: Difficult

INGREDIENTS

- 600g of bacon

- 2 lb pork shoulder

- ½ cup soy sauce

- ¾ cup hot sauce

- ½ cup ranch

DIRECTIONS

1. Bacon is first cooked and then make their small chops.

2. Add some ingredients like franks, sauce, and ranch dressing in a crockpot. Whisk them together, so they mix very well.

3. Then pour this mixture into a bacon crumble and put the pork into the crockpot.

4. Then allow it to heat at high pressure for four hours or at low up to 8 hours. on high for 4 hours or low 8 hours.

5. Freeze the pork and then serve it on bread sometimes; Pizza is also used.

NUTRITION: Calories: 91 kcal Fat: 7 g Protein: 3 g Carbs: 5 g

4. Pulled Pork Ofelia

Ready in: 6 hours 15 minutes

Servings: 5

Difficulty: Difficult

INGREDIENTS

- 3 lb pork shoulder

- 8 oz chopped onion

- ¾ cup wine

- 1 tbsp garlic paste

- ½ cup olive oil

- 2 tsp chopped thyme

- 2 tbsp coriander powder

- Black pepper to taste

- Salt to taste

- 2 tsp cinnamon

DIRECTIONS

1. Firstly, peel onions and make their small slices. Make tiny halves of garlic cloves. Mix these elements and soak them in the marinade. Take a freezer bag and add half of the onions to it.

2. Wash out the pork collar, make dry it, and shine it r with salt. Then put the pork collar in a freezer bag and soak it with marinade. Ensure there's no air in the bag and close it and position it in a mixing bowl. Then place the bowl in the refrigerator for 12 hours.

3. Turn on the oven and set its temperature at 125°C.

4. Then in an oven-specific dish, add meat onion mixture and marinade. Put this dish and heat it for 5-6hours. In a low cooker, meat is cooked in about 6-8 hours, and cooked meat will be very delectable.

5. It can be served with gravy.

NUTRITION: Calories: 758 kcal Fat: 59 g Protein: 40 g Carbs: 7 g

5. Stuffed Cabbage Rolls

Ready in: 80 minutes

Servings: 12

Difficulty: Difficult

INGREDIENTS

- ¼ cup water

- 1 lb ground beef

- One egg

- 1 tbsp onion powder

- 2 cups half cooked rice

- 26 oz Spaghetti sauce

- 1 tbsp garlic powder

- 1 cup Cabbage

- 1 tbsp black pepper

- 1 tbsp salt

DIRECTIONS

1. Take cabbage leaves, boil them for up to 4 mins, and put them in the cold water.

2. In a mixing bowl, add seasoning, ground beef, eggs, rice, and spaghetti, mix them all.

3. Place the ground beef mixture over the cabbage leaves one by the roll, then gently seal it with a toothpick.

4. In another pot, put spaghetti sauce, place the cabbage leaves, make another layer of spaghetti sauce, and a quarter cup of water simmer it for 1 hour at low flame.

5. Serve and enjoy it.

NUTRITION: Calories: 159.2 kcal Fat: 5 g Protein: 7 g Carbs: 25 g

6. Tofu and vegetable Satay Stir-fry

Ready in: 30 minutes

Servings: 5

Difficulty: Easy

INGREDIENTS

For the sauce

One diced red chili

1 tbsp peanut butter

Two diced garlic cloves

One juiced lime

Coriander leaves as required

2 tbsp ginger

1 tsp fish sauce

1 tbsp of soy sauce

- 1 tbsp yogurt

For stir-fry

- One diced leek

- 1 tsp coconut oil

- 2 cups noodles

- 400g firm tofu

- One diced pepper

- One diced carrot

- ½ diced of broccoli

DIRECTIONS

1. Put the ingredients of the sauce in a food processor and pulse it to make the sauce.

2. In a wok, add coconut oil and tofu and fry till it gets golden.

3. In another pan, boil the noodles according to packet details.

4. Now add vegetables in wok fry them but not lose the crunch of vegetables.

5. Add the sauce and stir it well. You may add water if required.

6. Add the noodles in wok and mix well.

NUTRITION: Calories: 97 kcal Fat: 7 g Protein: 1 g Carbs: 8 g

7. Spinach Russian Salad

Ready in: 40 minutes

Servings: 4

Difficulty: Medium

INGREDIENTS

- 4 tbsp olive oil

- Three tomatoes

- 200g block feta

- One minced garlic clove

- One diced green pepper

- Pitta bread to serve

- 1 tsp diced oregano

DIRECTIONS

1. Peel the tomatoes cut them into two pieces, scoop the seeds, now grate the seeds and the flash.

2. Season the tomatoes and do the scoping in a baking tray. Preheat the oven to 200 Fahrenheit.

3. Add cheese in garlicky tomatoes and cover them with tomato slices, oregano, salt, oil and chilies, and feta block. Bake it till it gets cooked.

NUTRITION: Calories: 243 kcal Fat: 21g Protein: 8 g Carbs: 4 g

8. Stovetop Spinach-Artichoke Dip

Ready in: 35 minutes

Servings: 5

Difficulty: Easy

INGREDIENTS

Bread bowl

- 1 Tbsp olive oil

- country loaf

- Salt to taste

Spinach-artichoke dip

- Black pepper to taste

- 1 tbsp unsalted butter

- 15 oz diced artichoke hearts

- One minced garlic clove

- 1 oz spinach

- 1 oz shredded cheese, parmesan

- Salt to taste

- Chips for serving

DIRECTIONS

1. Take the bread and make a hole in it to have a shape of bowl, now seasoned it with oil and salt and bake the bread for a half-hour

2. In a pan, add some butter and garlic fry. It nicely now adds artichokes spinach salt and stir it well.

3. In artichokes, add pepper parmesan and cream cheese till it gets melted.

4. Add the creamy sauce to the bread bowl, put some parmesan cheese over the top, and pepper bake it till it gets melted.

5. Enjoy the bread.

NUTRITION: Calories: 340 kcal Fat: 28 g Protein: 12 g Carbs: 10 g

9. Eggs in Purgatory

Ready in: 35 minutes

Servings: 4

Difficulty: Easy

INGREDIENTS

- 1/3 cup shredded cheese, parmesan

- 3 tbsp olive oil

- 2 tsp thyme, diced

- 1 ½ cups onion, diced

- ½ diced red pepper

- 9 oz artichoke hearts

- Salt to taste

- 28 oz smashed tomatoes

- Two smashed garlic clove

- 8 oz cubed potatoes

- Eight eggs

- 2 tbsp capers

DIRECTIONS

1. Take a large skillet with a good amount of oil, finely chopped onions, red pepper, add salt or taste, cook it for 10 mins.

2. Add diced tomatoes, chopped garlic, and artichokes in the pan and wait for simmer.

3. Add the boiled potatoes and capers in the skillet, mix it well with artichokes, season it with salt, and pepper sauce is ready.

4. In a glass baking dish, pour the artichokes sauce, make holes, and put the eggs in each of them.

5. Bake in the preheated oven around 350 Fahrenheit.

6. Enjoy the meal.

NUTRITION: Calories: 427 kcal Fat: 24.7 g Protein: 21.5 g Carbs: 5.7 g

10. Braised Artichokes with Tomatoes and Mint

Ready in: 30 minutes

Servings: 8

Difficulty: Easy

INGREDIENTS

- Two diced lemons

- 28 oz tomatoes

½ tsp chopped red pepper

1 ½ cups dry wine

2 tsp salt

12 anchovy fillets

1 cup olive oil

Eight minced garlic cloves

Six artichokes

1 cup mint leaves

DIRECTIONS

. Take crushed tomatoes in a large pot, season them with red pepper flakes, wine, salt, water, and oil.

. In a food processor, add artichokes and some cloves of garlic pulse it well. Now add coarse and half cup oil and pulse, make a perfect coarse pulse.

. Take light green leaves of artichokes, trim the stem with a knife. Rub the trimmed area with lemon. Scoop the artichokes with the help of a spoon, and rub the inner part with lemon.

. Make a layer of artichokes with past rubbing and merge in the crushed tomato mixture. Cook on medium flame, turn the artichokes from time to time.

. Now put the chokes in the plater and cover it with foil. Turn the flame high till the sauce get thickens. Add the sauce over chokes and enjoy.

NUTRITION: Calories: 370 kcal Fat: 28 g Protein: 6 g Carbs: 19 g

11. Tandoori Lamb Meatloaf

Ready in: 75 minutes

Servings: 4

Difficulty: Difficult

INGREDIENTS

- 1 lb Lamb

- Five cloves chopped Garlic

- One chopped onion

- One chopped Serrano pepper

- 2 tsp red chili

- 5 tbsp tomato paste

- ¼ tsp cinnamon

- 1 tsp coriander powder

- Salt to taste

- 1 tsp turmeric powder

- Black pepper to taste

- Two eggs

- ¼ tsp cloves

- 1 tbsp sliced mint

- ½ tsp Nutmeg

Topping

- 1 tsp garlic powder

- 5 tbsp tomato paste

- Salt to taste

- ¼ cup water

- Black pepper to taste

DIRECTIONS

1. Whisk all elements together in a mixing bowl and disperse the mixture in the oiled loaf pan.

2. Roast loaf at 350 F for 60 minutes.

3. Take a saucepan and add ingredients to it to make ketchup.

4. When the loaf is cooked, put ketchup on it and then again place it in the oven for 10 minutes.

5. Remove it from the oven stand it for 5 minutes to let it be cool.

6. Take the loaf out of the pan and serve it.

NUTRITION: Calories: 360 kcal Fat: 21 g Protein: 26 g Carbs: 17 g

12. Grilled Lemon and Rosemary Lamb chops

Ready in: 4 hours 25 minutes

Servings: 8

Difficulty: Difficult

INGREDIENTS

- ¼ tsp cinnamon

- ½ cup yogurt

- 1 tbsp chili

- 1 tbsp lemon juice

- Four cloves chopped Garlic

- 1 tsp Oregano

- 2 tbsp chopped rosemary

- Salt to taste

- Eight lamb

- ½ tsp black pepper

DIRECTIONS

1. Take a mixing bowl and mix rosemary, black pepper, lemon juice, salt, garlic, cinnamon, lemon zest, lemon zest, and yogurt in it. Take a large freezer bag and add lamb chops rinsed with marinade; Seal the bag and make sure there's no air in it. Put this bag in the refrigerator and freeze it for 4 hours.

2. Ready the grill for baking and oil it.

3. Place lamb chops soaked in a marinade, rinsed with salt and black pepper on a preheated grill, and bake it until chops are browned.

4. Heat them for about 3-4 minutes.

NUTRITION: Calories: 198 kcal Fat: 13.6 g Protein: 15.3 g Carbs: 4.5 g

13. Grilled lamb in Paleo Mint Cream Sauce

Ready in: 25 minutes

Servings: 5

Difficulty: Easy

INGREDIENTS

- 1/8 cup coconut milk

- One rack lamb

- ¼ cup crushed mint

- 2 tbsp crushed Dill

- 1 tbsp lemon juice

- 2 tbsp red chili

DIRECTIONS

1. Take a mixing bowl and blend all these ingredients.

2. Place this mixture in a refrigerator.

3. Take a lamb rack and marinate it with oregano and olive oil.

4. Store it at room temperature before baking.

5. Make grill ready at an appropriate heat that will be enough to cook lamb chops.

6. Put lamb chops on a hot grill and heat them for approximately 4 minutes.

7. Use tongs to flip the lamb approximately; it takes 4 minutes for the side and 8 for others to cook properly.

8. Dip lamb chops in sauce and enjoy.

NUTRITION: Calories: 267 kcal Fat: 11.3 g Protein: 36 g Carbs: 2 g

14. Spinach Lamb and Cauliflower Curry

Ready in: 75 minutes

Servings: 4

Difficulty: Difficult

INGREDIENTS

- 1 tsp peanut oil

- Two cloves chopped Garlic

- One crushed onion

- ½ cup curry paste

- 425 g sliced Italian Tomatoes

- 700 g sliced lamb

- 125 g crushed Spinach

- 1 ½ cups water

- 145 g chicken peas

- 350 g cauliflower

- Salt to taste

Crushed parsley

Black pepper to taste

DIRECTIONS

. Add the olive to a saucepan and heat it so that the pan is oil greased. Well, sliced onion and garlic are added and then stirred continuously for 1 minute until onions are softened. Then add a paste of curry, cook it, and stir until their fragrance comes out.

. Then add lamb and bake it and make sure all sides are browned. Later on, add water and tomatoes and boil them. Keep the intensity of heat varying from low to medium and medium to high. Cook it for about 45 minutes with continuous stirring. And then add chickpeas and cauliflower in it and cook and stir for about 5 minutes. Also, add spinach and stir it.

. Pour cooked spinach lamb and cauliflower curry in bowls and enjoy.

NUTRITION: Calories: 160 kcal Fat: 5.1 g Protein: 20.8 g Carbs: 7.8 g

5. Maple – Crusted Salmon Recipe

Ready in: 10minutes

Servings: 4

Difficulty: Easy

INGREDIENTS

1 tbsp red chili

2 tsp sugar

1 tbsp paprika

Salt to taste

- 3 tbsp maple syrup

- 1 ½ lb salmon fillets

DIRECTIONS

1. First, turn on the oven and heat it at a specific temperature.

2. Ingredients for this recipe are chili powder, paprika, sugar, and salt

3. Take a mixing cup and blend all these ingredients and make their mixture.

4. Take salmon fillets and spray them liberally with a mixture of chili powder. Place your salmon onto a prepared baking sheet & broil for 6 to 9 mins, dependent on how thick the fillets are & how crispy you prefer the crust.

5. Then place salmon over the aluminum baking sheet and broil it up to 6-10 minutes. Time for broiling can vary depending on personal interest.

6. Take out salmon from the oven and remove maple syrup present on the top of the salmon. Place it again in the oven and broil for about 12 more minutes, so that maple syrup is bubbled out. Now this Maple- the crusted salmon recipe is ready to serve.

NUTRITION: Calories: 300.21 kcal Fat: 11.29 g Protein: 34.27 g Carbs 14.1 g

Chapter 4: Snacks Recipes

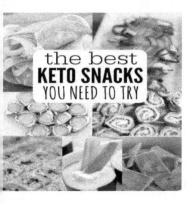

1. Baked mini–Bell Pepper

Ready in: 35 minutes

Servings: 5

Difficulty: Easy

INGREDIENTS

- 1 cup cheese

- 8 oz bell Pepper

- 1 tbsp chopped thyme

- 1 oz crushed chorizo

- 8 oz creamy cheese

- 2 tbsp olive oil

- ½ tbsp paprika paste

DIRECTIONS

1. Set your oven to 325 Fahrenheit.

2. Cut the bell peppers & remove all the core.

3. Combine the cream cheese, oil & spices in a container and mix in chorizo & herbs.

4. Place the mixture inside the empty bell pepper and sprinkle grated cheese.

5. Place the stuffed bell peppers in a baking tray sprayed with oil.

6. Bake in a preheated oven at 325 Fahrenheit for 18 minutes.

7. Serve and enjoy it.

NUTRITION: Calories: 411 kcal Fat: 38 g Protein: 12 g Carbs: 7 g

2. Caprese Snack

Ready in: 5 minutes

Servings: 5

Difficulty: Easy

INGREDIENTS

- Black pepper to taste

- 8 oz tomatoes

- 2 tbsp pesto

- 8 oz cheese

- Salt to taste

DIRECTIONS

1. Combine chopped tomatoes and diced cheese in a bowl.

2. Mix in pesto and toss well.

3. Sprinkle black pepper and salt to adjust the taste.

4. Serve and enjoy it.

NUTRITION: Calories: 218 kcal Fat: 16 g Protein: 14 g Carbs: 3 g

3. Caprese Bites

Ready in: 25 minutes

Servings: 5

Difficulty: Easy

INGREDIENTS

- Balsamic vinegar

- One sliced baguette

- Five chopped tomatoes

- 2 tbsp olive oil

- ½ cup crushed basil

- Salt to taste

- 12 oz chopped cheese

- Black pepper to taste

DIRECTIONS

1. Brush each bread slice with olive oil & put the slices in a baking tray.

2. Place the tray in a preheated oven set on the broiler and let it boil for four minutes.

3. Now add cheese slice and tomato slice followed by basil leaves and baguette slice over the broiled slice.

4. Drizzle with pepper and salt.

5. Bake in the preheated oven at 400 Fahrenheit for eight minutes.

6. Spread balsamic glaze and serve.

NUTRITION: Calories: 213 kcal Fat: 4 g Protein: 8 g Carbs: 36 g

4. Cauliflower Hash Brown

Ready in: 30 minutes

Servings: 12

Difficulty: Easy

INGREDIENTS

- ¼ tsp baking powder

- 1 lb cauliflower

- Two eggs

- 2 tbsp crushed onion

- ¼ tsp turmeric powder

½ cup cheddar, sliced

½ tsp garlic paste

Salt to taste

3 tbsp coconut flour

DIRECTIONS

. Grate the cauliflower in small pieces and add it to a bowl.

. Now, place the bowl in the microwave for three minutes.

. Spread the microwaved cauliflower over a paper towel for few minutes.

. Remove the maximum moisture out of the cauliflower.

. Add all the remaining ingredients in a bowl and cauliflower and mix well.

. Make tiny balls from the mixture and place the balls in a baking tray lined with butter paper.

. Bake in a preheated oven at 400 Fahrenheit for 15 minutes.

. Serve and enjoy it.

NUTRITION: Calories: 45 kcal Fat: 2.4 g Protein: 3.1 g Carbs: 3.4 g

. Sun-Dried Tomato Chicken Salad

Ready in: 25 minutes

Servings: 5

Difficulty: Easy

INGREDIENTS

- 1/3 cup of diced sun-dried tomatoes

- 2 cups of grated chicken, cooked

- 1/3 cup of mayonnaise

- 2 tbsp capers

- 2 tbsp parsley

- 2 tsp lemon juice

- Two onions, green

- ½ tsp black pepper

- ½ tsp salt

DIRECTIONS

1. In a medium mixing cup, combine all of the ingredients. To mix, sti
all together. Season with salt and pepper to taste.

2. Store in an airtight jar for up to five days.

NUTRITION: Calories: 386.6 kcal Fat: 20.8 g Protein: 24.6 g Carbs
20,1 g

6. Basic Crepes

Ready in: 30 minutes

Servings: 4

Difficulty: Easy

INGREDIENTS

- Two eggs

- 1 cup of all-purpose flour

- ½ cup of water

- ½ cup of milk

- 2 tbsp butter

- ¼ tsp salt

DIRECTIONS

1. Whisk the eggs & flour together in a wide mixing cup. Stir throughout the water or milk in a long, steady current. Combine the salt & butter in a mixing bowl and pound until smooth.

2. On medium to high flame heat frying pan or skillet. Using around 1/4 cup of batter per crepe, spill or shovel a batter on the griddle. Tilt the pan in some circular motion to uniformly brush the surface with batter.

3. Cook for around 2 mins, or until the bottom of the crepe is light brown. Turn, then cook another side after loosening with a spatula. Serve instantly.

NUTRITION: Calories: 216 kcal Fat: 9.2 g Protein: 7.4 g Carbs: 25. g

7. Whole-wheat Fettuccine with Kale and Goat's Cheese

Ready in: 45 minutes

Servings: 4.6

Difficulty: Medium

INGREDIENTS

- Salt to taste

- 2 tbsp olive oil

- Three diced onions, red

- 700 g lacinato kale, diced

- 340 g whole-wheat fettuccine

- Black pepper to taste

- 225 g goat cheese

Marinated Goat's Cheese

- 120 ml olive oil

- 225 g Goat's Cheese, diced

- ¼ tsp peppercorns

- Eight thyme sprigs

- Four bay leaves

- Three chopped garlic cloves

DIRECTIONS

1. Place the goat's cheese in the single-layer in a container to produce the goat's marinated cheese. Pour sufficient olive oil that fully coats the cheese along with garlic, thyme and bay leaf. Place it in the fridge until further use.

2. In such a wide frying pan on medium heat, melt the olive oil and add the pasta's onions. Cook for 10 minutes, or until the sides tend to brown. Add 1 tsp, reduce heat to medium-low, and simmer for another 15 to 20 minutes, or till onions are caramelized and soft.

Meanwhile, put some big pot of the water to a boil, then season generously with salt. According to the box directions, when the onions have caramelized, add the fettuccine to the boiling water & cook for 10-12 mins, or until al dente. Send the pasta to the pan after draining.

3. While the pasta is cooking, stir the kale into the onions, cover, then cook for 6-8 minutes, or until the kale is soft, stirring once maybe twice. Toss the pasta with the onion and kale combination, three-quarters of a marinated goat's cheese, and plenty of black pepper. Season to taste with a tbsp or more of the cheese's oil marinade. Serve warm with the crumble of leftover goat's cheese on top of each mug.

NUTRITION: Calories: 323 kcal Fat: 26.6 g Protein: 5.5 g Carbs: 16.5 g

8. Vegetarian Gumbo

Ready in: 60 minutes

Servings: 9

Difficulty: Medium

INGREDIENTS

- Two sliced red bell pepper

- ½ cup of butter

- 2/3 cup of all-purpose flour

- One chopped onion, white

- Two sliced celery stalks

- Five smashed garlic cloves

- 1 cup of okra, diced

- One diced cauliflower

- 3 cups of vegetable broth

- 14 oz tomatoes, toasted

- 1 lb. chopped mushrooms

- ½ tsp thyme, dried

- 2 tsp Cajun seasoning

- One bay leaf

- ½ tsp cayenne

- Pepper

- Salt

DIRECTIONS

1. Melt the butter over med to high heat in a bowl. In a different bowl, whisk together the flour & salt until well mixed. Cook for another 20 minutes, stirring continuously, or when the roux mixture achieves a rich amber-brown hue. Keep a careful watch on roux at all stages and should the fire if it appears to be cooked too fast or tends to smell burnt.

2. As soon as the roux is prepared, stir throughout the okra, bell peppers, onion, celery, & garlic until it is well mixed. Cook, stirring after 10 to 15 seconds, for another 5 minutes, or till these vegetables have softened.

3. Progressively whisk into vegetable stock till the broth is creamy. The cayenne, thyme, cauliflower, seasoning, onions, mushrooms, & bay leaf are then included. Stir until it is well mixed, then boil till the soup hits a simmer.

. Decrease the heat to almost medium to low and proceed to cook the umbo for another 5-10 mins, or till these vegetables are soft. If equired, season with additional salt, pepper, or/and cayenne.

. Serve directly over barley, served with a sprinkling of green nions. Please put it in the fridge for three days or freeze for three months until switching to a locked jar.

NUTRITION: Calories: 494 kcal Fat: 24.2 g Protein: 16.3 g Carbs: 56 g

. Potatoes Pancakes

Ready in: 20 minutes

Servings: 6

Difficulty: Easy

INGREDIENTS

- One egg

- Four potatoes

- One onion, yellow

- 2 tbsp all-purpose flour

- 1 tsp salt

- 2 cups of vegetable oil

- Black pepper

DIRECTIONS

1. In a broad mixing dish, finely grind the potatoes and onion. Every extra liquid should be extracted.

2. Combine the salt, egg, & black pepper in a mixing dish. Apply sufficient flour to thicken the paste, around 2-4 tbsp overall.

3. Preheat the oven to a low temperature of around 200 Fahrenheit.

4. Throughout the bottom of the heavy skillet, melt one-fourth-inch inch oil on medium to high heat. Through the hot oil, drop two to three one-fourth cup mounds and flatten and fry.

NUTRITION: Calories: 283 kcal Fat: 8.4 g Protein: 6.5 g Carbs: 46.7 g

10. Eggplant Gratin

Ready in: 60 minutes

Servings: 5

Difficulty: Medium

INGREDIENTS

- 13 cup bread crumbled

- Three diced eggplants

- 1 tsp Lemon Juice

- Four chopped tomatoes

- 1 tsp crushed thyme

- ¼ cup olive oil

- One bulb chopped garlic

- Salt to taste

- 4 oz cheese

- Black pepper to taste

DIRECTIONS

1. Combine tomatoes, salt, thyme, eggplant, olive oil, zest, pepper, and garlic in a bowl. Mix well.

2. To a baking tray, transfer the mixture & sprinkle goat cheese, panko, and olive oil over them.

3. In a preheated oven, bake it at 400 Fahrenheit for 55 minutes.

4. Serve and enjoy it.

NUTRITION: Calories: 302 kcal Fat: 24.3 g Protein: 9.4 g Carbs: 14 g

11. Cheesy Eggplant

Ready in: 45 minutes

Servings: 2

Difficulty: Medium

INGREDIENTS

- ½ cup tomato sauce

- Olive oil

- ¼ cup cheese

- ¾ lb Chopped eggplant

- Black pepper to taste

- One egg

- ½ cups chopped parmesan

- ¼ cup heavy cream

- Salt to taste

DIRECTIONS

1. At first, preheat your oven to 400 Fahrenheit.

2. Heat almost 1/8-inches of the olive oil in a large frying pan on med heat. When the oil is about smoking, you can add some slices of the eggplant & cook, turn once, till they're finely browned on sides & cooked thoroughly, about 5 mins. But be careful. It sometimes splatters. Shift those cooked slices of eggplant to thick tissue paper to drain it. Add some more oil, then heat & add some more eggplants till all of the slices have been cooked.

3. Meanwhile, in a small bowl, mix ricotta, half-&-half, egg, 1/8 tsp, 1/4 cups of Parmesan salt, & 1/8 tsp pepper.

4. In 2 separate gratin dishes, you have to place a layer of the eggplant slices & then sprinkle with the parmesan, pepper, salt & 1/2 spoon of marinara sauce. After that, add 2nd layer of the eggplant, more pepper & salt, half ricotta mixture, & at last 1 tbsp of the grated parmesan on its top.

5. Place gratins on a baking sheet & bake it for 25-30 mins or till that custard sets & its top is browned.

NUTRITION: Calories: 284 kcal Fat: 5.3 g Protein: 9.7 g Carbs: 24.1 g

12. Zucchini and Eggplant Gratin

Ready in: 20minutes

Servings: 4

Difficulty: Easy

INGREDIENTS

- 1/3 cup cheese

- Olive oil

- 25 oz diced zucchini

- 1 1/3 cup tomato sauce

- 370 crushed eggplant

DIRECTIONS

1. Preheat your non-stick pan on med heat. Then spray both the sides of zucchini & eggplant slices using some oil. Cook it in batches for

2 mins every side / till slightly browned & tender. Shift it to the plate. Then preheat your grill on med-high.

2. Layer 1/3 of zucchini, eggplant, sauce & cheese in the dish. Now repeat with the remaining eggplant, pasta sauce, zucchini & cheese.

3. Grill it for 5 mins / till cheese is melted & lightly browned.

NUTRITION: Calories: 746 kcal Fat: 10.2 g Protein: 10.8 g Carbs: 9.4 g

13. Brown Butter Cauliflower Mash

Ready in: 30 minutes

Servings: 6

Difficulty: Easy

INGREDIENTS

- 2 tbsp butter

- One crushed cauliflower

- Salt to taste

- ½ cup sour cream

- ½ tsp pepper

- 1 tbsp crushed chives

- ¼ cup chopped cheese

DIRECTIONS

. Fill water in the large oven to depth: 1/4 inch. Now arrange the cauliflower in the oven. Cover it while cooking on med-high heat for 7-10 mins / till tender. Then drain.

. Process the cauliflower, salt, pepper & sour cream in the food processor for 30 seconds - 1 min / till it's smooth, stop scraping down the sides as needed. Then stir in the Parmesan cheese & chives & place in a bowl.

. If wanted, put microwave mixture on HIGH for 1-2 mins/ till thoroughly heated, stir at 1-min intervals.

. Cook the butter in a small but heavy saucepan on med heat, constantly stirring, 4-5 mins / till the butter becomes golden brown. Then remove from the heat & immediately drizzle the butter on cauliflower mix. Garnish, if needed. Serve it immediately.

NUTRITION: Calories: 342 kcal Fat: 10 g Protein: 9 g Carbs: 5 g

4. Homemade Tortillas

Ready in: 30 minutes

Servings: 5

Difficulty: Easy

INGREDIENTS

3 tbsp olive oil

2 cups flour

¾ cups water

Salt to taste

DIRECTIONS

1. In the large bowl, mix flour & salt. Mix in water & oil. Turn it on the floured surface & knead it 10-12 times. Add some flour/water i desired to make a smooth dough. Then let it rest for 10 mins.

2. Divide the dough into eight pieces. On a lightly floured surface, ther roll each piece into a 7-inch circle.

3. Cook the tortillas on med heat till lightly browned, in the cast-iror pan, for 1 min on sides. Serve hot

NUTRITION: Calories: 159 kcal Fat: 5 g Protein: 3 g Carbs: 24 g

15. Red Cabbage Slaw

Ready in: 4 hours 15 minutes

Servings: 6

Difficulty: Difficult

INGREDIENTS

- 1 tbsp sugar

- One crushed Cabbage

- ½ cup mayonnaise

- ½ cup chopped carrot

- ¼ cup chopped cranberries

- 1 tbsp milk

- ¼ cups crushed walnuts

- 1 tbsp vinegar

DIRECTIONS

1. Mix cabbage, mayonnaise, carrot, cranberries, milk, walnuts, sugar, & cider vinegar in the bowl; mix well. Cover it & refrigerate till chilled, almost for 4 hrs.

NUTRITION: Calories: 216 kcal Fat: 18 g Protein: 2.4 g Carbs: 14 g

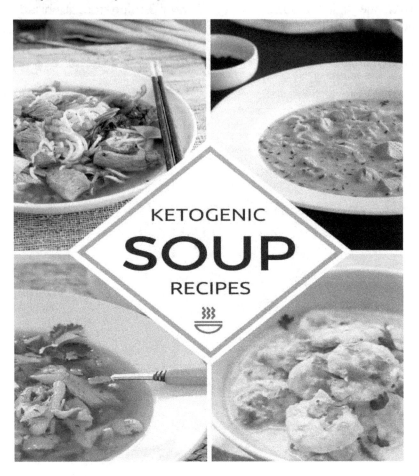

1. Harvest Pumpkin Soup

Ready in: 50 minutes

Servings: 8

Difficulty: Medium

INGREDIENTS

- 2 tbsp chopped pistachios

- 2 tbsp butter

- ½ chopped onion

- One chopped potato

- 4 ½ cups chicken soup

- Salt to taste

- 15 oz pumpkin puree

- ½ cup cream

- Black pepper to taste

- ¼ tsp nutmeg

- ½ cup milk

DIRECTIONS

1. In a cooking pan, mix onions and potatoes with butter for 9 to 11 minutes till the onion become translucent.

2. For fifteen minutes, boil it on low to medium flame.

3. Mix them in pumpkins until it becomes smooth; take salt and paper and the nutmeg to taste.

4. Cook it on high flame until it boils, and boil it for 9 to 11 minutes.

5. Mix it with milk and cream on flame, add salt and paper.

6. Serve it and enjoy it.

NUTRITION: Calories: 185 kcal Fat: 11 g Protein: 6 g Carbs: 17 g

2. Beef Stew

Ready in: 150 minutes

Servings: 4

Difficulty: Difficult

INGREDIENTS

- Two chopped potatoes, baking

- ¼ cup flour

- 1 lb beef

- ¼ tsp pepper

- 5 tsp oil

- 1 cup wine

- 2 tbsp vinegar

- 3 ½ cup beef coup

- One crushed onion

- Two chopped bay leaves

- Salt to taste

- Five chopped carrot

DIRECTIONS

1. Mix flour and pepper the beef and toss.

. In a pan, heat the oil and put pieces of beef one by 1. Cook it from all sides till brown color.

. In a pan, mix vinegar and wine and put them into the beef with beef broth and bay leaves. Boiled it until the beef become smooth and soft for about 90 minutes. Put carrots, potatoes, and onion in it and boil it for 25 to 30 minutes.

. Add water if it dries and flavors it with salt and pepper to taste and enjoy the meal.

NUTRITION: Calories: 494 kcal Fat: 2 g Protein: 35 g Carbs: 54 g

. Creamy Garlic Bacon Chicken Soup

Ready in: 30 minutes

Servings: 4

Difficulty: Easy

INGREDIENTS

2 tbsp crushed parsley

Four chopped bacon

Salt to taste

Six boneless chicken

Black pepper to taste

½ tsp garlic paste

8 oz chopped Mushroom

1 tsp chopped thyme

- ½ tsp onion powder

- One chopped onion

- ½ tsp sweet paprika

- Three cloves chopped Garlic

- 2/3 cup cream

- ¾ cup chicken soup

DIRECTIONS

1. In a pan, fry diced bacon until it becomes crispy.

2. Bake bacon pieces on the stove and set them on high flame. Flavo chicken thighs with garlic powder, pepper, paprika, salt, thyme, an onion powder.

3. Turn it and bake it from each side for 5 to 7 minutes on each side.

4. Add the onion to a frying pan and fry it for 120 seconds with garli in it with mushrooms for 20 seconds. Flavor them with salt an pepper to taste and cook it for 6 minutes; mix the chicken broth an mix it with cream and boil for 6 minutes.

5. Add chicken thighs to the front pan and cook it for 6 minutes till the source became thick.

6. Garnish it with bacon and parsley, serve it and enjoy it.

NUTRITION: Calories: 527 kcal Fat: 37 g Protein: 41 g Carbs: 8 g

4. Creamy Chicken Bacon Noodle Soup

Ready in: 45 minutes

Servings: 5

Difficulty: Easy

INGREDIENTS

- 1 oz egg noodles

- Six chopped bacon

- 1 tbsp Butter

- 1 lb chicken breast

- Three chopped ribs Celery

- Black pepper to taste

- One crushed onion

- 6 oz chopped Mushroom

- ½ tsp sliced thyme

- Two cloves chopped garlic

- Salt to taste

- 1 tsp garlic powder

- 4 cups chicken soup

- ½ tsp paprika

- 8 oz creamy cheese

- Chopped green onion

- 1 cup cream

- Crushed parsley

DIRECTIONS

1. In a frying pan, cook bacon till it becomes crispy.

2. Spread salt, garlic powdered, and black pepper on chicken breast.

3. Cook bacon and chicken breast for 180 seconds on each side.

4. Add one tablespoon butter to the frying pan; now mix onion, diced shallot, celery, and mushrooms till they become soft. Mix smoked paprika salt dried thyme, black pepper, garlic powder, and garlic, and cook it for 1 minute. Add

5. chicken stock which is 4 cups, and boil them. No mix in it, ramens, and egg noddle.

6. Add chicken and bacon to the pan mix and boiled for 16 minutes; also mix cream 1 cup cheese cubed and heavy cream when everything is fully mixed, then garnishes it with green onion, serve it and enjoy it

NUTRITION: Calories: 399 kcal Fat: 33 g Protein: 51 g Carbs: 47 g

5. Creamy Bacon Mushroom Thyme Chicken

Ready in: 35 minutes

Servings: 4

Difficulty: Medium

INGREDIENTS

- 1 tbsp thyme

- 4 lb boneless chicken

- Six chopped bacon

- 1 tbsp olive oil

- Salt to taste

- 1 tsp garlic powder

- 1 cup cream

- Black pepper to taste

DIRECTIONS

1. In a pan, mix chicken thighs and flavor them with salt and paper.

2. Cook chicken for 60 to 120 seconds till it becomes brown, and bakes them for 21 minutes in the oven until it is cooked.

3. Mix mushrooms with olive oil in a pan; now add thyme, began garlic powder has a cream salt and pepper. Boil it until the sauce becomes thick.

4. Mix chicken with them in the pan and cook it and serve the meal.

NUTRITION: Calories: 741 kcal Fat: 66 g Protein: 31 g Carbs: 6 g

6. Bacon Cheddar Ranch Chicken Noddle Soup

Ready in: 30 minutes

Servings: 5

Difficulty: Easy

INGREDIENTS

- 8 oz chopped cheese

- 1 tbsp olive oil

- 12 oz crushed bacon

- 1 cup crushed onion

- 8 cup chicken soup

- 1 oz Ranch Dressing

- 3 cup noodles

- 4 cups chicken, cooked

- 2 cups heavy cream (half and a half)

- ¼ cup chopped chives

DIRECTIONS

1. In a pan, add bacon pieces and fry until crispy over medium flame with occasional stirring. Drain and set aside.

2. In another pot, heat oil and sauté onions in it for more than five minutes.

3. Pour in chicken stock and let it boil.

4. Add noodles and cook for three minutes.

5. Add ranch dressing and a half and a half and whisk well.

6. Pour the ranch dressing mixture into the pot and mix well.

7. Mix in chicken and cook for few minutes.

8. Use cooked bacon, cheese, and chives for serving.

9. Enjoy it.

NUTRITION: Calories: 439 kcal Fat: 26 g Protein: 33 g Carbs: 19 g

. Rabbit Stew with Mushrooms

Ready in: 150 minutes

Servings: 4

Difficulty: difficult

INGREDIENTS

3 cups chicken soup

1 oz porcini Mushroom

1 tbsp olive oil

Three crushed shallots

Two chopped Garlic

1 ½ lb Mushroom

One rabbit

4 tbsp butter

2 cups Mushroom water

1 tbsp dried thyme

Salt to taste

One crushed parsnip

2 tbsp crushed parsley

DIRECTIONS

1. Soak the Mushroom in hot water and salt the rabbit pieces. In a ho
   oven, bake the garlic head drizzled with olive oil for ¾ hour.

2. Cut the rough end of mushrooms and dehydrate the porcini, and
   save the liquid of the mushrooms.

3. In a pan, release the water in mushrooms by heating them use sa
   for best results.

4. In a pan, add butter and rabbit pieces and cook it until the pieces
   became brown.

5. Put the shallots and cook it for 4 minutes, and spread the salt on
   also.

6. Now pinch the garlic in the water of Mushroom and mic them.

7. Combine the sherry or wine into the shallots, add mushroom and
   garlic mixture, and stir them.

8. Finally, add thyme, parsnips, Mushroom, and rabbit pieces, and mi:
   them well. And boil it for 1.5 hours

9. Sever it and enjoy it.

NUTRITION: Calories: 676 kcal Fat: 33.3 g Protein: 79.1 g Carbs: 21.
g

8. Rabbit Stew

Ready in: 70 minutes

Servings: 5

Difficulty: Medium

INGREDIENTS

- One crushed onion

- 4 Rabbit Legs

- Salt to taste

- 100 g flour

- Black pepper to taste

- 1 tbsp olive oil

- 25 g Butter

- One stick crushed celery

- 11 cup chicken stock

- 200 g mushroom

- One chopped Thyme

DIRECTIONS

1. Mix rabbit legs with a mixture of salt flour.

2. Bake the legs in butter and oil until the brown color is shown.

3. Combine the Mushroom, onion, and celery in a hot pot on medium flame. Combine flour with wine and mix with rabbit legs and also add thyme, chicken stock, and rabbit legs such that legs are merged in it.

4. Boil the mixture for up to 1-hour till tender the legs.

5. Serve It and enjoy the meal.

NUTRITION: Calories: 60 kcal Fat: 21 g Protein: 61 g Carbs: 36 g

9. Lentil and Sausage Soup Spinach Russian salad

Ready in: 3 hours 15 minutes

Servings: 10

Difficulty: Difficult

INGREDIENTS

- ½ lb Italian sausage
- One stalk Celery
- One crushed onion
- 16 oz Dry Lentils
- 1 tbsp garlic paste
- 1 cup chopped carrot
- 15.5 oz chicken soup
- 1 tbsp garlic powder
- 8 cups water
- 28 oz chopped tomatoes
- Two bay leaves
- 1 tbsp Crushed parsley
- ¼ tsp chopped Thyme
- ½ tsp Chopped Oregano

- ¼ tsp Chopped basil

- Salt to taste

- ½ lb pasta

- Black pepper to taste

DIRECTIONS

1. Add sausage to a pan and cook it till brown and mix the onion, celery, sauté, and garlic.

2. Combine carrot, tomatoes, water, chicken broth in lentils.

3. Flavor them with pepper, oregano, thyme, garlic powder, salt, bay leaves, and basil.

4. Boil the mixture for 150 to 180 minutes till lentils become soft. Now add pasta and bake it for 18 to 19 minutes.

NUTRITION: Calories: 353 kcal Fat: 8 g Protein: 18.9 g Carbs: 50.2 g

10. White Chicken Chili

Ready in: 15 minutes

Servings: 6

Difficulty: Easy

INGREDIENTS

- 14.5 oz chicken soup

- One chopped onion

- Two cloves chopped Garlic

- 1 tbsp olive oil

- 1 ½ tsp cumin

- ½ tsp paprika

- ½ tsp chopped coriander

- ¼ tsp Cayenne pepper

- ½ tsp chopped oregano

- Salt to taste

- 7 oz green pepper

- 8 oz cheese

- 15 oz cannellini beans

- One ¼ cup corn

- 2 ½ cup chopped Rotisserie, cooked

- 2 tbsp crushed Cilantro

- 1 tbsp Lemon juice

- Tortilla chips

DIRECTIONS

1. In oil, mix onion and garlic and cook it.

2. Mix cumin, cayenne pepper, green chilies, oregano, chicken broth, and paprika; add the salt and pepper flavor and boil it for 16 minutes.

. Drain the beans, add them to the blender, process them with broth, and puree until soft and smooth.

. Mix the cheese and corn with beans and processed beans, mix them, and boil for 9 to 10 minutes. Finally, mix lime juice and cilantro.

. Serve and enjoy it,

UTRITION: Calories: 383 kcal Fat: 14 g Protein: 33 g Carbs: 35 g

1. Keto Crab Dip Soup

eady in: 15 minutes

ervings: 6

ifficulty: Easy

INGREDIENTS

1 lb Lump crabmeat

1 tbsp ghee

¾ cup Chopped Parmesan Cheese

Tbsp seasoning

3 cups milk (Half and Half)

8 oz cream cheese

DIRECTIONS

in a pan, add butter and cream cheese, whisk, stir and smooth it. Mix parmesan cheese using a blender or mixer until it becomes smooth, softly put crab meat, avoid chunks, and finally, the soup is ready to enjoy.

NUTRITION: Calories: 358 kcal Fat: 27 g Protein: 21 g Carbs: 5 g

12. Tomato Feta soup

Ready in: 30 minutes

Servings: 6

Difficulty: Easy

INGREDIENTS

- 2/3 cup chopped Cheese

- 2 tbsp butter

- 1/3 cup cream

- ¼ cup crushed onion

- 3 cups water

- Two cloves chopped Garlic

- 1 tsp sugar

- Salt to taste

- 1 tsp honey

- Black pepper to taste

- Ten crushed tomatoes

- 1 tsp pesto sauce

- ½ tsp chopped oregano

- 1 tbsp tomato paste

- 1 tsp crushed basil

DIRECTIONS

1. in olive oil, mix onion and cook for 120 seconds, garlic for 1 minute. Now combine tomatoes, water, salt, basil, pepper, oregano, pesto, boil them, and add sweeteners. Bake it for 20 to 25 minutes. Finally, using a blender made it smooth and also mixed cream and cheese in it. Serve and enjoy it.

NUTRITION: Calories: 170 kcal Fat: 13 g Protein: 4 g Carbs: 10 g

13. Creamy Keto Tuscan Soup

Ready in: 17 minutes

Servings: 6

Difficulty: Easy

INGREDIENTS

- 1 cup chopped spinach

- 1 lb sausage

- 1 cup cream

- Two stalks chopped celery

- ¼ cup chopped Garlic

- 3 cup beef soup

- 8 oz cream cheese

- 1 cup red chili

DIRECTIONS

1. In a pan, brown the sausage and break it into pieces. Set sausages aside. In the same pan, add onions and celery and cook until soft add garlic and cook for 3 minutes. Mix sausages back to the pot and add cream cheese and roasted red peppers. Mix until cheeses are melted into meat and vegetables. Stir and add beef stock and bring it to boil. Remove heat and add cream while whisking it. When spinach is soft, and soup is cooked. Remove it from flame and serve

NUTRITION: Calories: 534 kcal Fat: 23 g Protein: 17 g Carbs: 9 g

14. Creamy Tuscan Garlic Tortellini Soup

Ready in: 15 minutes

Servings: 8

Difficulty: Easy

INGREDIENTS

- 2 cups chopped spinach

- 2 tbsp butter

- 9 oz tortellini

- One chopped onion

- 4 cups chicken soup

- 2 cup chopped chicken, cooked

- 28 oz chopped tomatoes

  Black pepper to taste

  1 cup cream

- Salt to taste

- 1 tbsp Italian seasoning

- ¼ cup chopped parmesan cheese

DIRECTIONS

1. In a pan, heat the butter and combine onion, and garlic and bake it. Put chicken broth, salt and pepper, diced tomatoes, Italian seasoning, white beans, parmesan cheese, and heavy cream in it and boil it. Combine the chicken, tortellini, and spinach and boil for 12 minutes till it thickens.

NUTRITION: Calories: 397 kcal Fat: 20 g Protein: 21 g Carbs: 34 g

15. Keto Smoked Sausage Cheddar Beer Soup

Ready in: 6 Hours 30 minutes

Servings: 14

Difficulty: Difficult

INGREDIENTS

- 2 cups cheddar Cheese

- 8 oz cheese cream

- 14 oz Beef

- 1 cup cream

- 12 oz beer (extra Beef Soup)

- Black pepper to taste

- 1 cup crushed Carrots

1 cup crushed celery

Salt to taste

One chopped onion

1 tsp Red chili

Four cloves chopped garlic

IRECTIONS

in cooked, combine celery, salt and pepper, sausage, garlic, beef stock, red pepper flakes, and onion and cook for 3 to 4 hours. Then mix cream, cheddar, and cream cheese. Mix it well using a blender or whisk it well. Add salt and pepper if needed and bake it for more time. Serve and enjoy it.

UTRITION: Calories: 244 kcal Fat: 17 g Protein: 5 g Carbs: 4 g

Chapter 6: Salad Recipes

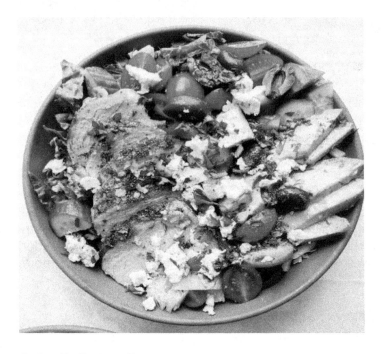

1. Garlic Broccoli

Ready in 5 minutes

Servings: 3

Difficulty: Easy

INGREDIENTS

- 2 tbsp lemon juice

- 1 ½ cup Broccoli florets

- 1 tbsp olive oil

- Black pepper to taste

- 1 tbsp butter

- Three garlic cloves

- salt to taste

DIRECTIONS

1. Boil the broccoli for 1-2 minutes. Drain and keep aside.

2. Take a skillet and heat over medium flame. Put butter and oil in it and fry garlic till it is brown.

3. Now add broccoli.

4. Season with salt and pepper and add lemon juice.

5. Stir well and remove from stove.

6. Serve and enjoy.

NUTRITION: Calories: 111 cal Fat: 8 g Protein: 2 g Carbs: 7 g

2. Creamed Coconut Spinach

Ready in 25 minutes

Servings: 3

Difficulty: Easy

INGREDIENTS

- Black pepper to taste

- 3 tbsp of ghee

- Two shallots

- 20 oz spinach leaves

- 1 tbsp minced ginger

- ½ tsp of cumin

- 2 tbsp of jalapeno chile

- 1 cup of coconut milk

- salt to taste

- 2 tbsp of all-purpose flour

DIRECTIONS

1. Heat ghee in a large Dutch oven and cook spinach for 3-5 minutes. Drain and keep aside to cool. Then chop it.

2. Melt 2 tbsp of ghee in a pan over medium heat. Cook jalapeno, ginger, and shallots for 3-5 minutes. Add cumin, sugar, and flour and cook for 2-3 minutes.

3. Add coconut milk and whisk well.

4. Bring a boil and allow it to simmer for 2-3 minutes.

5. Add chopped spinach.

6. Season with salt and pepper.

7. Serve and enjoy.

NUTRITION: Calories: 139.2 kcal Fat: 9.2 g Protein: 2.6 g Carbs: 12.1 g

3. Creamed Cauliflower

Ready in 10 minutes

Servings: 8

Difficulty: Easy

INGREDIENTS

- Black pepper

- 2 ½ cups Cauliflower

- Three garlic cloves

- 1 tsp of parsley

- One diced onion

- 1/4 cup butter

- ¼ cup all-purpose flour

- 1 cup whole milk

- ½ cup of parmesan cheese

DIRECTIONS

1. Steam, drain and cool the cauliflower.

2. Melt butter in the skillet and add flour. Cook till it forms a paste.

3. Add garlic and onion and cook at high heat.

4. Add milk slowly.

5. Stir continuously till the cream is formed.

6. Season with salt and pepper.

7. Mix the cheese in it and stir till it is melted.

8. Add cauliflower and allow to simmer for 3-5 minutes.

9. If the sauce is too thick, add milk according to the requirement.

10. Garnish with parsley and pepper.

11. Serve and enjoy.

NUTRITION: Calories: 176k cal Fat: 4 g Protein: 4 g Carbs: 7 g

4. Radishes with Herbed Salt and Olive Oil

Ready in: 25 minutes

Servings: 8

Difficulty: Easy

INGREDIENTS

- 1 tsp of salt

- Two garlic clove

- 2tbsp of chopped parsley

- 1 tsp of olive oil

- 2tbsp of chopped chives

- 1tbsp of chopped tarragon leaves

- ½ tsp of peppercorns

- 2tsp of grated lemon zest

- 2 lb of radishes

DIRECTIONS

Mix all the ingredients in a large bowl.

Season with salt and pepper.

Add oil in a separate small bowl.

Serve radishes with herbed salt and oil for dipping.

Enjoy.

NUTRITION: Calories: 83, Fat: 12 g, Proteins: 1 g, Carbs: 4 g

Grilled Asparagus Medley

Ready in: 25 minutes

Servings: 8

Difficulty: Easy

INGREDIENTS

¼ tsp of dill weed

1 lb asparagus

1 cup sliced mushrooms

2 cups pepper (Yellow, red, and green)

¼ tsp pepper

One chopped tomato

2tbsp of olive oil

One garlic clove

1tsp of parsley

- ½ tsp of salt

- ¼ tsp of lemon pepper

DIRECTIONS

1. Mix vegetables, garlic, and olives in a bowl.

2. Add oil and toss to coat.

3. Sprinkle it with parsley, pepper, salt, and lemon pepper.

4. Toss again well.

5. Grill over medium heat for 20-30 minutes.

6. Stir occasionally.

7. Serve and enjoy.

NUTRITION: Calories: 78 cal Fat: 5 g Protein: 3g Carbs: 8 g

6. Creamy Fennel Sauce

Ready in: 20 minutes

Servings: 6

Difficulty: Easy

INGREDIENTS

- Salt to taste

- 2 cups Cream

- One shallot

- ½ cup White wine

- One garlic clove

- 2 tbsp White flour

- 1 oz cream cheese

- ½ tsp Herbs

- White pepper to taste

- 2 tbsp nutmeg, grated

DIRECTIONS

1. Take a food processor and process chopped shallot and fennel till they are minced completely.

2. Take a pot and melt butter. Add vegetables and cook for 2-5 minutes.

3. Now transfer cooked vegetables to a separate bowl and keep them aside.

4. Melt butter and add flour to it.

5. Cook till it becomes golden.

6. Add white wine. Stir continuously.

7. Add cream and cheese and cook till it melts.

8. Return vegetables to pot and mix with sauce, herbs, and nutmeg.

9. Season with salt and pepper. Simmer for 15-20 minutes.

10. Serve and enjoy.

NUTRITION: Calories: 200 cal Fat: 8 g Protein: 10 g Carbs: 20 g

7. Zucchini with Mint

Ready in: 15 minutes

Servings: 4

Difficulty: Easy

INGREDIENTS

- 1 tbsp of mint, chopped

- 12 small zucchini

- 2 Scallions

- 2 tbsp olive oil

- 1 tbsp lemon juice

- Salt to taste

- ½ tbsp of parsley leaf, chopped

DIRECTIONS

1. Cut zucchini lengthwise.

2. Take a skillet and heat olive oil over medium heat.

3. Add scallions and sauté.

4. Add zucchini and salt to taste.

5. When zucchini starts to become golden, then reduce the heat.

6. Add lemon juice and sprinkle mint & parsley.

7. Cook for 1-2 minutes.

3. Serve and enjoy.

NUTRITION: Calories: 125 cal Fat: 8 g Protein: 5 g Carbs: 13 g

3. Warm Crab and Spinach Dip

Ready in: 20 minutes

Servings: 2

Difficulty: Easy

INGREDIENTS

- 2 cups cheddar cheese

- 2tbsp olive oil

- Two minced garlic cloves

- 1/3 cup chopped onion

- 1 cup cream cheese

- ¼ cup of milk

- 1 cup garlic and herb cheese

- ¼ cup wine

- 2 tsp of Worcestershire sauce

- 1 tbsp of seafood seasoning

- 1/8 tsp of red pepper flakes

- 2 cups chopped spinach

- 2 lb crabmeat

- Tortilla chips

DIRECTIONS

1. Take a skillet and heat over medium flame.

2. Cook onion and garlic for 2-3 minutes.

3. Add cheese and Boursin and stir till melted.

4. Add cream, wine, and milk.

5. Stir continuously.

6. Add seasonings and remaining ingredients.

7. Cook till cheeses are melted.

8. Serve and enjoy.

NUTRITION: Calories: 170 cal Fat: 14g Protein: 9 g Carbs: 2 g

9. Okra Gumbo

Ready in: 15 minutes

Servings: 8

Difficulty: Easy

INGREDIENTS

- 2 Bay leaves

- One chopped onion

- One garlic clove

One chopped bell pepper

8 oz sliced mushrooms

Two okra

½ tsp of file powder

One diced tomatoes

3 tbsp of vegetable oil

1 tsp of salt

1 tsp of black pepper

2 tbsp of all-purpose flour

DIRECTIONS

1. Take pan and heat oil in it over medium heat.

2. Add garlic, bell pepper, and onion.

3. Sauté till tendered.

4. Add mushrooms, tomatoes, tomato paste, file powder, okra, ba
    leaves, salt & pepper.

5. Stir continuously and cook for 35-40 minutes.

6. Take 2 tbsp of oil in the pan and heat over medium flame. Add flou
    and cook for 3-5 minutes till it becomes golden.

7. Add roux in okra mixture and cook for 5-10 minutes till it i
    thickened.

8. Serve and enjoy.

NUTRITION: Calories: 105 cal Fat: 5.5g Protein: 3.2 g Carbs: 12.4 g

10. Stuffed Mushrooms

Ready in: 25 minutes

Servings: 12

Difficulty: Easy

INGREDIENTS

- ¼ tsp of onion powder

- 12 mushrooms

- 1 tbsp minced garlic

- 1 tbsp of vegetable oil

- 1 cup Cream cheese

  ¼ tsp of black pepper

  ¼ cup of parmesan cheese

  ¼ tsp of cayenne pepper

DIRECTIONS

1. Take a large skillet and heat oil.

2. Add garlic and mushrooms' stems.

3. Fry till all the moisture is absorbed. Keep aside and let it cool.

4. Once the mixture is cooled at room temperature, add parmesan and cream cheese, cayenne pepper, onion powder, and black pepper.

5. The mixture should be thick.

6. Fill the mushrooms with the mixture.

7. Arrange the mushrooms in a baking dish.

8. Bake for 15-20 minutes.

9. Serve and enjoy.

NUTRITION: Calories: 88 cal Fat: 8.2 g Protein:2. 7 g Carbs: 1.5 g

11. Seattle Asian Salmon Bowl

Ready in: 10 minutes

Servings: 4

Difficulty: Easy

INGREDIENTS

- One strip Shredded nori

- ½ cup green onions

- 1tbsp sesame seeds (toasted)

- One sliced English cucumber

- 2 cups rice cooked

- 14 oz diced avocado

- ¾ cup Daikon radish

- Salt to taste

- 16 oz salmon

- Black pepper to taste

DIRECTIONS

1. Take a large bowl and mix vinaigrette ingredients.

2. Take a pan and spray with oil.

3. Season the salmon and heat for 4-5 minutes.

4. Divide the hot rice into four bowls.

5. Top with green onions, sesame seeds, cucumbers, sprouts, and avocado.

6. Put salmon in each bowl.

7. Drizzle with vinaigrette.

8. Sprinkle with nori.

9. Serve and enjoy.

NUTRITION: Calories: 395 cal Fat: 5 g Protein:27 g Carbs: 31 g

2. White Bean and Cod Salad

Ready in: 25 minutes

Servings: 3

Difficulty: Easy

INGREDIENTS

4 tbsp olive oil

300 g white beans

- One diced carrot

- One diced spring onion

- One garlic clove

- Apple cider vinegar as required

- Salt to taste

- Chives as required

DIRECTIONS

1. Take white beans in a pot. Add water till it is covered.

2. Add salt (one pinch) and let it boil for 10-20 minutes.

3. Drain and keep aside.

4. Simmer water in a pot. Put cod in it and cook for 5-10 minutes.

5. Process the garlic in the food processor.

6. Blend oil, vinegar, and garlic. Pour this mixture over cod.

7. Add carrot (shredded) to the beans.

8. Layer the beans on the plate. Divide the cod on top of each plate and sprinkle chives (chopped).

NUTRITION: Calories: 1439 cal Fat: 106.7 g Protein: 68.1 g Carbs: 54.7 g

13. Three Herb Tomato Zucchini Salad

Ready in: 10 minutes

Servings: 4

ifficulty: Easy

IGREDIENTS

1 cup Chopped herbs (chive, parsley, basil)

2 cups cherry tomatoes

One sliced shallot

One zucchini

2 tbsp of lemon juice

4 tbsp Virgin oil

1 tsp Garlic

2 tsp Sumac

Smoked paprika

1 tbsp of lemon juice

salt to taste

pepper to taste

1 Lemon slices round

DIRECTIONS

1. Slice tomatoes and zucchini and put in a large bowl.

2. Slice and soak the shallot in lemon juice. Keep aside.

3. Toss together the chopped herbs in a separate bowl.

4. Mix olive oil, sumac, garlic, salt, lemon juice, pepper, paprika in large bowl.

5. Add tomatoes and zucchini.

6. Add shallot slices and herbs.

7. Toss well.

8. Garnish with lemon slices.

9. Serve and enjoy.

NUTRITION: Calories: 84 cal Fat: 8.8 g Protein: 0.5 g Carbs: 1.9 g

14. Spinach and Cabbage Slaw

Ready in: 10 minutes

Servings: 6

Difficulty: Easy

INGREDIENTS

- ¼ tsp of dried weed
- 2 cups coleslaw
- ¼ cup red bell pepper
- 2 cups spinach leaves
- ¼ cup ranch salad dressing

DIRECTIONS

1. Mix all the ingredients in a large bowl.
2. Keep in the refrigerator for 10-15 minutes.
3. Serve and enjoy.

NUTRITION: Calories: 35 cal Fat: 20 g Protein: 2 g Carbs: 3 g

5. Avocado Bell Pepper Salad

Ready in: 5 minutes

Servings: 1

Difficulty: Easy

INGREDIENTS

Two sliced onions

One diced avocado

½ cup cherry tomatoes

- One diced bell pepper

- 2 tbsp of parsley (minced)

- Salt to taste

- 2 tbsp Lemon juice

- Black pepper to taste

DIRECTIONS

1. Mix all the ingredients in a large bowl.

2. Refrigerate for 5-10 minutes.

3. Serve and enjoy.

NUTRITION: Calories: 391 cal Fat: 30 g Protein: 7 g Carbs: 34 g

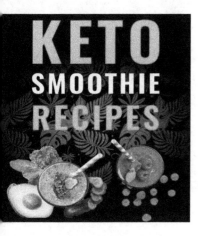

1. Spinach and Avocado Smoothie

Ready in: 3 minutes

Servings: 1

Difficulty: Easy

INGREDIENTS

- 1 cup cold water

- 1 cup chopped mango, frozen

- 2 cups baby spinach

- ½ avocado

- 2 tbsp protein powder

DIRECTIONS

1. Combine mango, spinach, protein powder, avocado, and water in a food processor and blend to get a smooth mixture.

2. Transfer the into the serving glass.

3. Serve and enjoy it.

NUTRITION: Calories: 329 cal Fat: 17 g Protein: 17 g Carbs: 44 g

2. Café Latte

Ready in: 15 minutes

Servings: 4

Difficulty: Easy

INGREDIENTS

- 1 1/3 cup coffee

- 2 cups milk

DIRECTIONS

1. Add milk to the pan and let it boil with constant vigorous stirring to form foam in heating milk.

2. Add coffee to a container and pour in hot water. Stir to dissolve coffee in water.

3. Transfer the coffee into serving cups.

4. Add boiling milk in serving cups and stir

Serve and enjoy it.

UTRITION: Calories: 63 cal Fat: 2.5 g Protein: 4.7 g Carbs: 5.7 g

Hot Chocolate

eady in: 6 minutes

ervings: 4

ifficulty: Easy

IGREDIENTS

¼ tsp vanilla extract

4 cups milk

¼ cup sugar

¼ cup cocoa powder

½ cup chocolate chips

RECTIONS

Add sugar with cocoa and milk in a pan and heat on medium flame with constant stirring.

Stir in chocolate chips and mix to dissolve them.

Mix in vanilla extract and stir well.

Serve and enjoy it.

JTRITION: Calories: 323 cal Fat: 13 g Protein: 9 g Carbs: 42 g

4. Strawberry Protein Smoothie

Ready in: 10 minutes

Servings: 1

Difficulty: Easy

INGREDIENTS

- Five ice cubes

- ½ cup almond milk

- One vanilla protein

- ¾ cup strawberries

- ½ cup greek yogurt

- 1 tsp honey

DIRECTIONS

1. Add all the ingredients into the blender except for ice cubes and blend to get a smooth mixture.

2. In the end, add ice cubes and blend again.

3. Serve and enjoy it.

NUTRITION: Calories: 304 cal Fat: 9.1 g Protein: 31.7 g Carbs: 21.6

5. Avocado Raspberry and Chocolate Smoothie

Ready in: 5 minutes

Servings: 1

Difficulty: Easy

INGREDIENTS

- ½ tsp vanilla

- ½ avocado

- 1 tbsp maple syrup

- 1 ½ cups milk

- 1 cup raspberries

- 1 tbsp cocoa powder

DIRECTIONS

1. Add all the ingredients to a food processor and blend to get a smooth, creamy mixture.

2. Serve and enjoy it.

NUTRITION: Calories: 360 cal Fat: 14 g Protein: 10 g Carbs: 55 g

Berry Coconut Chia Smoothie

Ready in: 5 minutes

Servings: 2

Difficulty: Easy

INGREDIENTS

- 1 tbsp maple syrup

- 1 cup mixed berries

- One ¼ tbsp coconut milk

- Seven ice cubes

- 1 tbsp chia seeds

- 1 tbsp toasted coconut flakes

DIRECTIONS

1. Soak chia seed in milk and leave it for 20 hours.

2. Add all the ingredients to a food processor and blend to get a smooth, creamy mixture.

3. Serve and enjoy it.

NUTRITION: Calories: 133 kcal Fat: 8 g Protein: 3 g Carbs: 16 g

7. Orange Creamsicle Smoothie

Ready in: 5 minutes

Servings: 2

Difficulty: Easy

INGREDIENTS

- One sliced orange

- One sliced banana

- ½ cup orange juice

- 2 tsp vanilla extract

- ¾ yogurt

DIRECTIONS

1. Add all the ingredients to a food processor and blend to get a smooth, creamy mixture.

2. Serve and enjoy it.

NUTRITION: Calories: 207 kcal Fat: 2 g Protein: 3 g Carbs: 24 g

3. Mint Cocoa Mix

Ready in: 5 minutes

Servings: 53

Difficulty: Easy

INGREDIENTS

- Miniature marshmallows

- 1 cup creamer

- 7 ½ cups chocolate drink

- 2 ½ cups sugar

- 2 oz milk powder

- 25 peppermint candies

DIRECTIONS

1. Add sugar, milk powder, candies, and marshmallows in an airtight bag and shake well.

2. Add cocoa mix and hot milk in a container and stir.

3. Add marshmallows and serve.

NUTRITION: Calories: 259 cal Fat: 9 g Protein: 14 g Carbs: 42 g

9. Chicken Misco Soup

Ready in: 5 minutes

Servings: 2

Difficulty: Easy

INGREDIENTS

- 1 cup spinach

- 2 cups water

- 2 tbsp ginger

- One garlic clove

- 120 sliced chicken

- Two diced mushrooms

- One sliced zucchini

- 2 tbsp miso paste

DIRECTIONS

1. Add water to a pot and let it boil.

2. Stir in garlic and ginger and cook for few minutes.

3. Add chicken pieces and mix. Bring it to simmer for five minutes.

4. Mix in Mushroom and zucchini and cook for five more minutes.

5. Add miso paste and spinach. Cook for one minute.

Serve and enjoy it.

NUTRITION: Calories: 134 cal Fat: 3.1 g Protein: 19 g Carbs: 8.5 g

Conclusion

In some studies, the keto diet has been shown to increase energy balance mood, control blood sugar, improve cholesterol, lower blood pressure, and much more. For intractable epilepsy, the keto diet is successful and reasonably safe treatment choice. Despite its long history, much remains unknown about the diet, including its modes of operation, the right care, and its applicability range. Diet trials provide useful insight into the causes of seizures and epilepsy and the possible therapies that could be needed. However, if the diet is used incorrectly it may have serious health consequences and may not be the best way to achieve and maintain optimal health. It takes the body around two weeks, and sometimes four weeks, to adjust to the drastic reduction of carbohydrates.

In general, the ketogenic diet has unique effects on the body and cells providing benefits that far outweigh those offered by nearly any other diet. The combination of carbs restriction and ketone production reduces insulin levels, stimulates autophagy (cell cleaning), increases mitochondrial chemical growth and efficiency, lowers inflammation, and burns fat. High-fat and the low-carb diet must be prevented during breastfeeding, pregnancy, infancy, and rehabilitation from medical conditions. If you're unsure whether the Keto diet is right for you, seek advice and help from the doctor. It is crucial to talk to a dietitian, doctor, or other trustworthy healthcare professional before starting new diet, particularly if someone is trying to treat a health condition or illness. To guarantee that the keto diet is a healthy eating pattern, people interested in beginning it should meet with a doctor to check whether they have heart disease, diabetes, hypoglycemia, or other medical conditions.

Please remember that there aren't many reports on the ketogenic diet long-term benefits. It's uncertain if following this diet for a longer time more productive than following less restrictive healthy eating habits.